Precision Medicine in Cardiovascular Disease Prevention

AF379082

Seth S. Martin

Editor

Precision Medicine in Cardiovascular Disease Prevention

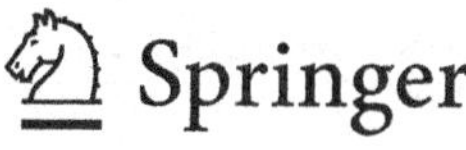 Springer

Editor
Seth S. Martin
Digital Health Innovation Laboratory,
Ciccarone Center for the Prevention of
Cardiovascular Disease, Division of
Cardiology, Department of Medicine
Johns Hopkins University School of
Medicine, Johns Hopkins Hospital
Baltimore, MD, USA

ISBN 978-3-030-75057-2   ISBN 978-3-030-75055-8   (eBook)
https://doi.org/10.1007/978-3-030-75055-8

© Springer Nature Switzerland AG 2021
This work is subject to copyright. All rights are reserved by the Publisher, whether the whole or part of the material is concerned, specifically the rights of translation, reprinting, reuse of illustrations, recitation, broadcasting, reproduction on microfilms or in any other physical way, and transmission or information storage and retrieval, electronic adaptation, computer software, or by similar or dissimilar methodology now known or hereafter developed.
The use of general descriptive names, registered names, trademarks, service marks, etc. in this publication does not imply, even in the absence of a specific statement, that such names are exempt from the relevant protective laws and regulations and therefore free for general use.
The publisher, the authors and the editors are safe to assume that the advice and information in this book are believed to be true and accurate at the date of publication. Neither the publisher nor the authors or the editors give a warranty, expressed or implied, with respect to the material contained herein or for any errors or omissions that may have been made. The publisher remains neutral with regard to jurisdictional claims in published maps and institutional affiliations.

This Springer imprint is published by the registered company Springer Nature Switzerland AG
The registered company address is: Gewerbestrasse 11, 6330 Cham, Switzerland

Preface

Welcome to "Precision Medicine in Cardiovascular Disease Prevention". The uniquely comprehensive book was made possible by tapping into the diverse and talented faculty at the Johns Hopkins Ciccarone Center for the Prevention of Cardiovascular Disease. Faculty members involved junior colleagues in chapters, which is essential not only to bringing fresh perspectives to the topic, but also to building the future leaders of precision medicine.

Preventive Cardiology is a proactive, patient-centered, and multidisciplinary team-oriented medical subspeciality dedicated to mitigating cardiovascular risk through research, education, and the highest level of clinical care tailored to a patient's risk profile. The field of Preventive Cardiology uses lifestyle interventions and evidence-based medical treatments to prevent the onset of cardiovascular disease in people at risk and to prevent further issues in people who already have cardiovascular disease.

Prevention can be initiated earlier or later in the course of disease. Primordial prevention is preventing risk factors for cardiovascular disease in the first place. Primary prevention is preventing cardiovascular events. Secondary prevention is about preventing subsequent events after an initial event has already occurred. All are important and will be addressed in this book.

With a view towards cardiovascular disease prevention, this book aims to provide a comprehensive, forward-thinking, and inspiring take on precision medicine. It is infused with ample opinion informed by the best science to date and establishes fundamental principles that regardless of the rapid advances in technology will remain timeless guiding forces. While the focus is on use of precision medicine in cardiovascular disease prevention, many of the learnings are relevant and important to other areas of medicine.

Precision medicine has varied definitions. The US Food and Drug Administration defined precision medicine as "an innovative approach to tailoring disease prevention and treatment that takes into account differences in people's genes, environments, and lifestyles." This definition is particularly comprehensive and captures the movement to a tailored approach from a one-size-fits-all approach. Related terms often include personalized medicine and individualized medicine.

Cardiovascular disease prevention is especially well suited for precision medicine. The field is naturally forward looking, aiming to getting ahead of the curve by predicting the future and averting problems before they happen using the latest evidence-based innovations. This involves stopping the progression of atherosclerosis in its tracks and preventing cardiovascular events like heart attacks and strokes before they occur and cause devastating consequences. Preventive cardiology is an area with vigorous research activity on the cutting-edge of precision medicine topics. The field has traditionally focused on population-based approaches, with more recent movement towards precision medicine, and the tension between these is interesting to explore.

Frequently the discussion of precision medicine takes on a narrower focus limited to genomics or targeted pharmaceuticals. However, the opportunity for precision medicine is much larger, as highlighted in this book. While genes, molecules, and novel pharmaceuticals are key components of precision medicine, viewing precision medicine through only this lens would be analogous in the preventive cardiology world to focusing only on one risk factor that contributes to atherosclerotic cardiovascular disease. To harness the potential, we must be comprehensive.

As such, the topics in this include:

- Social Determinants of Health
- Biomarkers
- Genomics
- Atherosclerosis Imaging
- Digital Health
- Machine Learning / Artificial Intelligence
- Novel Research Methodologies
- Shared Decision-Making

The book's 3 large aims are to:

1. Plot the path of precision medicine in cardiovascular disease prevention
2. Review advanced precision medicine techniques and their potential in the future
3. Establish the ground rules for the evaluation of new prevention techniques

Precision medicine is at an exciting intersection. It opens up new data streams, new ways to process these data, and new ways to empower patients, their caregivers, and clinicians with these data. It also opens up new ways to test if interventions work.

This book begins with a focus on social determinants of health because all of the work that we do in precision medicine must be viewed through the lens of health equity. Through this lens, we acknowledge that the most vulnerable in our society need tailored tools to level the playing field. It is essential that research in this area is diverse and inclusive. To this end, the national Precision Medicine Initiative changed its name to "All of Us", reflecting the critical value of diversity and inclusion in precision medicine.

A common goal of precision medicine has been, "the right treatment for the right patient at the right time". This emphasizes treatment as the ultimate impact of precision medicine. This is appropriate, in that ultimately what matters is what we can do to take action to help. But precision medicine is not only about treatment. It is about diagnostics, even pre-diagnostics, screening, and prevention too. And diagnostic and contextual data from new sensors, lab tests, and imaging, can play a key role in informing treatment.

This book comes at a critical time in cardiology and in medicine. The concept of precision medicine is not new, but we have new tools to realize the potential of precision medicine. The digital age is disrupting medicine and it's happening so rapidly that no one can fully keep up or know exactly where it's going. However, clearly we are moving to a future of precision medicine where everything revolves around the patient. A lot must align to deliver the right care to the right patient at the right time. We are talking about moving from the population average to notable subgroups to the individual. We are talking about moving from one-size-fits-all approaches to tailored approaches.

Precision medicine brings together the fields of mobile and digital health, big data, genetic medicine, and artificial intelligence. As precision medicine approaches lead us to understand the individual better, we will understand the individual earlier in life, at the edge of wellness, such that future disease is predicted and prevented. But how do we make this a reality? It starts with understanding the pieces that are in this book.

It is hoped that you will return to key sections of this book as you move forward in your own journey applying the principles of precision medicine to build the health care system of the future. Meanwhile, you may find that as additional studies and discoveries emerge, the foundation of this book will provide a solid footing to understand and apply new findings.

It is anticipated that the book will be updated from time to time, to incorporate the latest concepts and advances. Your feedback is most welcomed. If there are certain topics that you would like to see covered in future editions of this book, please email smart100@jhmi.edu.

Baltimore, MD, USA   Seth S. Martin

Acknowledgments

Building a textbook from scratch is no short order. This first edition of *Precision Medicine in Cardiovascular Disease Prevention* was possible because of a large amount work and effective collaboration of many individuals. I would like to thank the wonderfully supportive staff at Springer. In particular, Mr. Grant Weston worked closely with me in his role as Executive Editor to plan this book and get it off the ground. A huge thanks is also due to Mr. Suresh Rettagunta, whose tireless work as Project Coordinator kept us moving forward and brought this book to the finish line. This book is made possible by the incredible team of authors who were generous enough to lend their time and expertise, working off a blank page to bring this book to the world. Finally, I thank my wife, Nguyen, and son, Asher, for their love and support. Over Asher's first decade of life, I have a great deal of hope that we will make tremendous progress in building a world that harnessing the science of precision medicine for healing around the globe.

Contents

Social Determinants

Zulqarnain Javed, Hashim Jilani, Tamer Yahya, Safi U. Khan, Prachi Dubey, Adnan Hyder, Miguel Cainzos-Achirica, Bita Kash, and Khurram Nasir

Social Determinants of Health and Cardiovascular Care: A Historical Perspective

Dr. Martin Luther King Jr. once said, "Of all the forms of inequality, injustice in healthcare is the most shocking and inhumane." These words are as relevant today as nearly 60 years ago, when they were first spoken by Dr. King at a convention of the Medical Committee for Human Rights in Chicago in March of 1966 [1]. As elusive as the concept of health equity sounds, inequities in health and healthcare

Z. Javed · M. Cainzos-Achirica · B. Kash
Center for Outcomes Research, Houston Methodist, Houston, TX, USA

H. Jilani
Department of Medicine, Carle Foundation Hospital, Urbana, IL, USA

T. Yahya · P. Dubey
Houston Methodist Hospital. Houston Methodist Research Institute, Houston, TX, USA

S. U. Khan
West Virginia University, Morgantown, WV, US

A. Hyder
Milken Institute School of Public Health, George Washington University, Washington, DC, US

M. Cainzos-Achirica · K. Nasir (✉)
Division of Cardiovascular Prevention and Wellness, Department of Cardiology, Houston Methodist DeBakey Heart & Vascular Center, Houston, TX, USA
e-mail: khurram.nasir@yale.edu

K. Nasir
Center for Computational Health and Precision Medicine, Houston Methodist, Houston, TX, USA

Division of Health Equity and Disparities Research, Center for Outcomes Research, Houston, TX, USA

© Springer Nature Switzerland AG 2021
S. S. Martin (ed.), *Precision Medicine in Cardiovascular Disease Prevention*,
https://doi.org/10.1007/978-3-030-75055-8_1

are explained—to a large extent—by the conditions in which individuals live and work, procreate and grow old, form social networks, and seek and provide help [2]. These conditions—collectively known as the social determinants of health (SDOH) —determine our physical, emotional and financial wellbeing, susceptibility to illness, and overall health and quality of life [3] (Fig. 1).

Traditional models of health and medical care in the US have historically ignored the role of SDOH in predicting wellness and illness [4]. However, radical changes in healthcare financing in the past decade, including performance-based reimbursement mechanisms such as value-based care models, coupled with the documented benefits of primary and secondary prevention on healthcare expenditures and overall value of services, have highlighted the importance of acknowledging and incorporating SDOH in chronic disease prevention and management [5, 6]; these changes in healthcare financing and overall service delivery have helped bring SDOH to 'mainstream' clinical practice models, including care for cardiovascular disease (CVD) [5–7].

SDOH provide unique opportunities for tailoring medical care to the individual patient, thereby improving health outcomes and reducing observed disparities by informing equitable resource utilization and health services delivery [8–10]. Despite the proven link between SDOH and health outcomes, and the demonstrated urgency to incorporate SDOH into existing and any future policy and practice models, social determinants are grossly under-utilized—to the detriment of the individual patient, and the population at large [4, 11]. In particular, current frameworks of 'precision care' rarely incorporate SDOH into clinical decision management tools, severely limiting the documented benefits of SDOH application in clinical settings [9, 12, 13].

Fig. 1 Social determinants of health

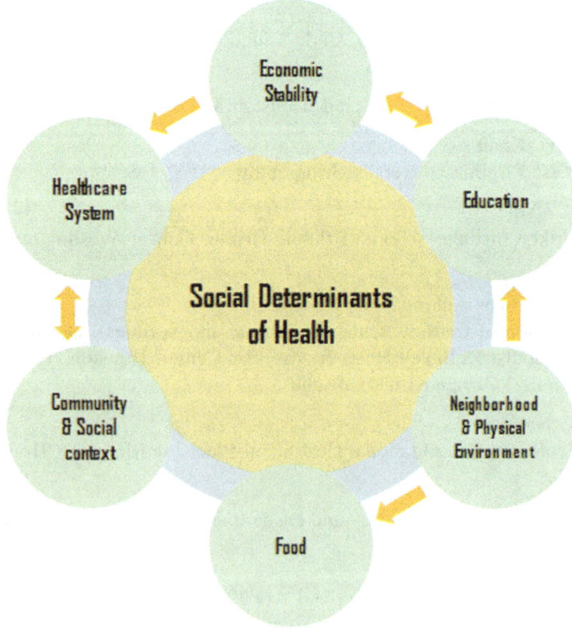

President Barack Obama launched the Precision Medicine Initiative in 2015, and outlined its goals as, '…delivering the right treatments, at the right time, every time to the right person' [14]. However, recent evidence points to the challenges and shortcomings of contemporary precision medicine—from both an economic and health outcomes perspective—owing to inattention to SDOH [13, 15, 16]. Indeed, real-world evidence clearly suggests that SDOH integration into clinical care is associated with improved outcomes in vulnerable populations [17, 18]. Consequently, novel health services delivery approaches advocate for the use of individuals' unique social and environmental *risk factor* profile to guide disease prevention and management efforts and maximize the utility of *precision health*, with major implications for health equity [12, 15].

This chapter discusses SDOH in the context of disparities in CVD care and outcomes. We highlight the link between different SDOH domains and CVD; potential role of SDOH in identifying high-risk, marginalized population subgroups; and the use of SDOH knowledge to inform care delivery to underserved populations, given their unique SDOH burden. In addition, we provide a brief overview of the major efforts in highlighting disparities in health and healthcare in the US over the past four decades.

Landmark Reports on Health Disparities: Relevance to CVD

Much awareness, attention and work in the field of health disparities and minority health is pioneered by the landmark report on minority health, "Black and Minority Health", issued in 1985 by then Secretary of US Health and Human Services, Margaret M. Heckler [19]. The critical report presented objective evidence of wide disparities in health outcomes, experienced disproportionately by the minority populations in the US, particularly the Black population. The Heckler report was the first detailed account of health disparities on a national level in the US, and the first major acknowledgement of such disparities by the US government. The report highlighted that heart disease and stroke were the leading cause of excess mortality in Black people compared to White people—with an average annual excess mortality burden of 31% [19].

It was not until nearly two decades later that the findings from the Hecker report were used as a framework to build on work in the field, and determine future directions on a path to health equity. The groundbreaking Institute of Medicine (IOM) report titled "Unequal Treatment: Confronting Racial and Ethnic Disparities in Healthcare," [20] analyzed evidence from nearly 600 published studies and revealed glaring racial/ethnic disparities in outcomes for major medical conditions, including CVD. The IOM report provided the first comprehensive framework to address disparities in health and healthcare, with a particular focus on race, racism, and discrimination, and the interplay of various SDOH to produce health outcomes in minority populations. The report concluded with a set of recommendations, and provided a basis for design of interventions to address such disparities—a framework that many academicians, clinicians, population health scientists and policy makers have used in the past two decades.

Subsequently, the American College of Cardiology (ACC) and the Henry J. Kaiser Family Foundation (KFF) published a joint review of disparities in cardiovascular services in the US, and reported that Black people were less likely than White people to receive diagnostic and revascularization procedures, even after adjusting for patient characteristics [21].

These accounts were followed by major work from the Centers for Disease Control and Prevention (CDC): "State of Health Disparities and Inequalities in the US," [22] and two landmark scientific statements on SDOH from the American Heart Association [23, 24]. These reports further acted as stark reminders of the fact that healthcare in the US in general, and cardiovascular care specifically, are not equitable, and that much needed attention must be accorded to SDOH if the goals of health equity were to be achieved nationally. These reports are summarized in Table 1.

Prior work presents important opportunities to further knowledge on health disparities in the US, including frameworks that can—and must—be used to design evidence-based, scientifically robust interventions in order to address various SDOH and improve CVD risk and outcomes in vulnerable populations. The goal is to inform future actions to incorporate SDOH into policy-making and clinical practice, and reduce disparities in CVD and associated outcomes locally, nationally and globally.

Role of SDOH in Cardiovascular Care: Ignored for Far Too Long

Current State of CVD Disparities in the US

CVD is the leading cause of death in the US, [25] with significant financial implications for both patients and the healthcare system. The cost of CVD in the US is estimated at nearly $550 billion annually, including $237 billion in lost productivity due to premature CVD and stroke [26]. By 2035, the direct costs associated with CVD are expected to double in the US, with nearly 45% of the population expected to develop some form of CVD [26]. Marginalized populations, such as racial/ethnic minorities are affected disproportionately by CVD, and its risk factors [27–29].

Recent data from Centers for Disease Control and Prevention (CDC) [27] show that non-Hispanic Black people experience nearly 1.5 times increased prevalence of hypertension and diabetes, and 20% higher rates of CVD related mortality, relative to non-Hispanic White people. Non-Hispanic Black people are more than twice as likely to die from heart disease, compared to other minority groups, including non-Hispanic Asian people or Pacific Islanders. While a decreasing trend in CVD

Table 1 Landmark reports on health disparities in the US

Agency	Published	Title	Major CVD related findings	Link
U.S Department of Health and Human Services. *Contributor: Heckler, M*	1985	Report of the Secretary's Task Force on Black & Minority Health. The 'Heckler' Report	Heart disease and stroke were the leading cause of excess mortality in the Black population, compared to their White counterparts	https://collections. nlm.nih.gov/ catalog/nlm: nlmuid-8602912- mvset
Institute of Medicine (US) Committee on Understanding and Eliminating Racial and Ethnic Disparities in Health Care *Smedley, BD. et al*	2002	Unequal Treatment: Confronting Racial and Ethnic Disparities in Healthcare	Black people were less likely to undergo cardiac catheterization, revascularization procedures or CABS after MI, compared to White people	https://www.nap. edu/catalog/ 12875/unequal- treatment- confronting-racial- and-ethnic- disparities-in- health-care
Henry J. Kaiser Family Foundation. *Lillie-Blanton, M. et al*	2002	Racial/Ethnic Differences in Cardiac Care: The Weight of the Evidence	Black people were less likely than White people to receive diagnostic and revascularization procedures, even after adjusting for patient characteristics	https://www.kff. org/wp-content/ uploads/2002/09/ 6040r-racial-and- ethnic-differences- in-cardiac-care- report.pdf
Centers for Disease Control and Prevention: State of Health Disparities and Inequalities in the US	2013	CDC Health Disparities and Inequalities Report	Age-adjusted coronary heart disease (CHD) death rate was higher among non-Hispanic Black people than any other racial/ ethnic group. Rate of premature death (aged < 75 yrs) was higher among non-Hispanic Black people than their White counterparts	https://www.cdc. gov/ minorityhealth/ CHDIReport.html

prevalence is observed in non-Hispanic White people over the past two decades, rates of heart disease have remained relatively unchanged in racial/ethnic minority populations [27].

Such disparities are linked to multiple SDOH in underserved populations—including barriers to care and socioeconomic disadvantage—which exert both independent and cumulative effects on CVD outcomes. For example, rates of most CVD preventive services are higher in non-Hispanic White people, relative to other racial/ethnic groups [27, 30]. Compared to non-Hispanic White people, Asian people are reported to have 60–64% lower likelihood of routine weight and blood pressure screening, whereas Hispanic people are over 50% less likely to report routine blood pressure measurement, and 66% less likely to be asked by their healthcare provider about smoking habits [30].

A recent study of nearly 45,000 non-institutionalized US adults reported substantial and persistent disparities in CVD prevalence by socioeconomic status (SES), from 1999–2016 [31]. Abdalla et al. found that overall prevalence of congestive heart failure (CHF) and stroke was less than one-third, and less than one-half in the 'highest resource' group, respectively, relative to the remainder of the population. In addition, disparities in CVD prevalence between the highest and lowest resource groups have widened over the past twenty years [31].

SDOH are important predictors of disparities in CVD risk and outcomes, and are particularly relevant to CVD prevention and management [23]. Current models of CVD care are mostly designed to address *traditional* risk factors for CVD; much effort, energy and resources have been allocated to the *medical determinants of health* [32]. However, past and present models of CVD care seldom acknowledge the critical role of SDOH, or the failure of leaders in the field to build a comprehensive yet personalized care model, informed by SDOH. Meaningful reductions in cardiovascular health disparities cannot be achieved without incorporating SDOH into existing models of care, and informing CVD prevention and management approaches. Indeed, SDOH are critical to achieving true equity in cardiovascular care, and outcomes.

SDOH, 'Traditional' Risk Factors and Current Models of CVD Care

Most existing practice models of CVD prevention target traditional *downstream* CVD risk factors such as cigarette smoking, diabetes mellitus, obesity, hypertension and physical activity; [33] very few recognize SDOH as major *upstream* determinants of CVD outcomes, and fewer yet, identify potential mechanisms to incorporate SDOH into prevention efforts—both on a policy and practice level [32, 33]. Contrary to current norms of CVD care, years of research have shown that a 'prescription' for healthy behaviors seldom achieves the intended goal of lower CVD risk, or improved clinical outcomes in most patients [34–36]. Instead, improvements in individual risk factor profile require a multi-faceted approach that targets different SDOH domains, as well as pathways that link each domain to CVD outcomes [32, 33].

Addressing *upstream* determinants of health is a top Healthy People 2030 goal: "creating social, physical, and economic environments that promote attaining the full potential for health and well-being for all" [37]. It is known that medical care for traditional disease risk factors accounts for only 10–20% of the variation in health outcomes; the rest is explained by our behaviors, environment, and the conditions in which we live and work, i.e. SDOH [38]. Indeed, findings from a unique population-based study using data from over 3000 US counties across 45 states demonstrate that socioeconomic factors, health behaviors, medical care and physical environment contribute 47, 34, 16 and 3%, respectively to a composite health outcomes score on a national level in the US [36].

Equitable healthcare resource distribution, such as uniform access to best practice interventions for CVD prevention can significantly reduce disparities risk in CVD mortality, overall and by SES [39]. However, current best practices rarely incorporate SDOH as the "causes of causes," i.e. upstream determinants of classic CVD risk factors—a missed opportunity for population health management. Unfortunately, improvements in CVD care have not been shared equally among different population subgroups over the past century. Indeed disparities in CVD risk and outcomes persist across a wide spectrum of SDOH [29, 31, 40, 41]. As discussed in the following sections, SDOH affect CVD not only directly but also indirectly via effects on health behaviors and other traditional risk factors. These pathways are discussed in greater detail in the following sections.

SDOH and CVD: A Review of Current Literature

The link between individual socioeconomic factors and health outcomes has been extensively studied. However, relatively few studies have investigated the association between different SDOH domains and risk factors, overall burden and long-term outcomes for CVD.

The landmark American Heart Association (AHA) "Scientific Statement on Social Determinants of Risk and Outcomes for Cardiovascular Disease" highlighted major shortcomings of the US healthcare system in failing to address, and incorporate SDOH into policies and practices for cardiovascular care [24]. The report also highlighted critical knowledge gaps that must be filled in order to move the needle from health disparity to health equity; particularly if we are to stem the rising burden of CVD in the US, which continues to impact marginalized populations disproportionately, and is projected to rise to over 45% by 2035—a 30% increase since 2015 [26].

The following subsections review existing knowledge of the link between different SDOH—organized into distinct domains and subdomains—and CVD. Each section discusses current evidence and major pathways of the SDOH-CVD link.

SDOH: A Domain-Based Analysis

SDOH influence CVD via multiple pathways and mechanisms. The association between SDOH within each domain and CVD, and possible pathways of the observed association are discussed briefly in this section. As depicted in Fig. 1, SDOH do not act in isolation; rather different SDOH interact to influence CVD. The discussion of SDOH herein is based on the frameworks proposed by Healthy People 2020 and the Kaiser Family Foundation, [2, 42] which organize SDOH into six distinct domains: economic stability, education, food, neighborhood and physical environment, health care system and community and social context.

Economic Stability

Economic stability is defined by income, wealth, employment status and occupational category. While other definitions of economic stability also include physical living conditions, education and food insecurity, [2, 42] those are discussed separately, given their independent association with CVD. This section focuses on income and employment as the major measures of economic stability.

Current Evidence and Pathways

The association between low income and increased risk of myocardial infarction (MI), heart failure and stroke is seen across study designs and target populations [43, 44]. In a unique computer simulation study of over 31 million US adults aged 35–64 years, Hamad et al. [45] analyzed the association between low SES (defined as <150% of federal poverty level [FPL] or education less than high school) and premature (i.e. occurring before age 65 years) CHD and myocardial infarction (MI) deaths, and found that rates of premature MI and CHD mortality were twice as high in the low SES group, relative to high SES group. The authors further demonstrated that SES-associated 'upstream' risk factors explained a greater proportion of the observed mortality disparities, compared to traditional risk factors (60% vs. 40%, respectively).

A meta-analysis of 70 studies reported an overall increased risk of acute myocardial infarction (AMI) for all three measures of SES, i.e. income, education and occupation [46]. The study found 71% increased AMI risk for low income (pooled relative risk [RR] 1.71; 95% CI 1.43–2.05); 34% for low education (pooled RR 1.34; 95% CI 1.22–1.47); and 35% for low occupational socioeconomic position (pooled RR 1.35; 95% CI 1.19–1.53). Another meta-analysis of over 50 studies reported an increased risk of hypertension associated with socioeconomic adversity [47]. Leng et al. found 19% (pooled odds ratio [OR] 1.19; 95%

CI = 0.96–1.48), 31% (pooled OR 1.31; 95%CI 1.04–1.64) and over 100% (pooled OR 2.02; 95%CI 1.55–2.63) increased risk of hypertension for income, occupation and education, respectively.

These findings are further corroborated by results from the landmark Whitehall study of nearly 18,000 British civil servants, which showed that civil servants in the lowest SES category had nearly 3 times increased risk of CHD mortality over a 10-year period, compared to those in the highest SES category; smoking and other traditional CVD risk factors only explained part of the observed mortality difference [48].

The association between economic stability and population level CVD outcomes has been analyzed on a global scale. For example, in a comprehensive review of published literature on SES and stroke outcomes, Addo et al. [49] reported that both stroke mortality and disability-adjusted life years (DALY) lost are over threefold higher in low income countries, compared to high and middle income countries. A national prospective cohort study of over 45,000 patients in Netherlands, followed for three years, reported a 37–39% increased relative risk of AMI and 55–74% increased relative risk of chronic ischemic heart disease (CIHD), with the variation attributed to gender [50]. Similarly, the Atherosclerosis Risk in Communities (ARIC) study—a large-scale, prospective cohort of nearly 10,000 community-dwelling, predominantly black and white men and women—found that participants who experienced decline in income levels over a mean follow-up of 17 years had higher risk of MI and stroke, compared to those whose income remained relatively unchanged [51]. Conversely, participants whose income increased during the study period experienced lower incidence of CVD compared to those individuals whose income was unchanged [51].

Employment status and occupational category are important markers of economic stability, and independent determinants of CVD. Unemployment, change in employment status, blue collar/service occupational categories and job stress are all linked to poor CVD outcomes in a variety of target populations. For example, a unique prospective study of over 40,000 Japanese men and women followed for an average of 15 years reported a 1.5–threefold increased risk of stroke incidence and stroke mortality in individuals who experienced job loss (Hazard Ratio [HR] for stroke incidence, men 1.58 [95%CI 1.18–2.13]; HR for stroke mortality, women 2.48 [95%CI 1.26–4.77]) or reemployment (HR for stroke incidence, men 2.96 [95%CI = 1.89–4.62]; HR for stroke mortality, women = 2.48 [95%CI = 1.26–4.77]) [52].

In addition to the direct effects on CVD, economic stability plays a major role in determining a variety of CVD outcomes via indirect effects on other SDOH domains. Multiple proposed mechanisms link SES and CVD; most of which are based on the interplay of different SDOH domains potentiating the risk of adverse CVD outcomes. For example, loss of income has been associated with consumption of unhealthy foods, unhealthy behaviors such as smoking, and greater degree of psychological stress and depression, which are in turn linked to elevated risk of CVD [53, 54]. Income level and loss of employment can affect health insurance coverage, access to medical care and neighborhood of residence; all of which impact cardiovascular health [55]. Higher SES facilitates access to resources such as knowledge, social networks, safe/stable housing and access to health care that can mitigate the negative effects of economic instability on CVD and overall health [56].

Summary

- *Economic stability affects CVD through a multitude of direct and indirect pathways, with great implications for both individual and population cardiovascular health*
- *CVD treatment and prevention efforts must carefully consider the role of economic stability, both on a clinical and policy level*
- *Future research must focus on development and validation of an exhaustive measure of economic stability, inclusive of income and wealth, education, and occupational status and employment, to be applied to diverse population subgroups*

Education

The association between education and health, wellbeing and quality of life is well documented in the literature [57]. Education impacts health broadly, and CVD in particular, via numerous pathways. The discussion of education herein includes both formal educational attainment, and health literacy.

Current Evidence and Pathways

Low educational attainment is associated with adverse CVD risk factor profile and increased risk of CVD incidence and mortality [41]. Results from the recent Prospective Urban Rural Epidemiologic (PURE) study of over 150,000 participants from 20 countries globally—followed for an average of 7.5 years—document a 1.23 to 2.23 times increased risk of major cardiovascular events for low educational attainment, relative to high level of education, with the highest risk observed in low-income countries (HR [low vs high level of education] 2.23; 95% CI 1.79–2.77). These results are supported by a meta-analysis of 72 cohort studies from Asia, Europe and the US, which reported an up to 40% higher risk of stroke, CAD and cardiovascular mortality in individuals with low educational attainment, relative to their counterparts [58].

INTERHEART—a case–control study of over 26,000 participants from 52 countries reported an over 30% increased risk of non-fatal AMI associated with less than 8 years of education; the observed association persisted even after adjusting for a variety of sociodemographic and clinical covariates [59, 60]. Similarly, findings from the ARIC study—a prospective study of 13,948 White and African American adults aged 45–64 years—demonstrated an inverse relationship between educational attainment and lifetime CVD risk; [61] Kubota et al. found that over 1 in 2 participants with less than high school education experienced a lifetime event of CVD.

Education can affect CVD outcomes both directly and indirectly via effects on other SDOH. In general, academic success is linked to higher earnings, which in turn provide resources for access to healthcare, better housing and healthier food options [62–64]. Further, education is an important determinant of occupational status; low educational attainment is linked to unemployment, which predisposes to poverty, food insecurity, unstable/unsafe housing and various other intermediary behavioral and environmental factors that predict adverse CVD outcomes [65].

Nearly 80 million U.S adults are reported to have limited health literacy, which is associated with poor health outcomes [66]. Higher education levels increase access to, and understanding of, important resources such as recommendations/ guidelines for a balanced diet, physical activity, as well as available evidence on risk factors, prevention and management of major chronic illnesses, including CVD [67].

It has been previously reported that individuals with limited health literacy are more likely to adopt unhealthy behaviors such as smoking, and less likely to achieve cessation [68, 69]. The negative effects of education on adverse CVD outcomes such as coronary artery disease (CAD) persist, regardless of other sociodemographic factors and clinical predictors [70]. Conversely, higher health literacy is associated with healthy behaviors, positive lifestyle changes, and increased medication adherence [71, 72].

Traditional risk factors such as diabetes, hypertension and body mass index (BMI) have been shown to mediate the relationship between education and CVD [122], which further reinforces the intersectional nature of SDOH, i.e. effects on cardiovascular health via multiple direct and indirect pathways, including inter-linkages among different SDOH domains, as well as between each domain and traditional/clinical risk factors.

Summary

- *Education exerts important influences on cardiovascular health, both directly and indirectly via 'facilitatory' effects on other SDOH such as income and occupation*
- *Education—both formal educational attainment and health literacy—play an important role in shaping our behaviors, and determining the risk of CVD*
- *Future efforts must focus on elucidating possible pathways between education and various upstream and downstream CVD risk factors*
- *Effects of education and other SDOH, including income, occupation and race/racism must be analyzed from an intersectionality lens*

Neighborhood and Physical Environment

This diverse domain encompasses various aspects of housing (e.g. safety, quality), physical environmental conditions such as air/water quality, availability of playgrounds, greenness, walkability, availability of hospitals, schools and grocery stores, and public transport [2]. Our built environment determines access to a wide range of other SDOH, and factors that can directly or indirectly affect risk of CVD. For example, neighborhood safety and sidewalk availability to facilitate physical activity and availability of nearby hospital to receive immediate medical care. These relationships and pathways linking neighborhood/physical environment to both CVD, and other SDOH, are discussed below.

Current Evidence and Pathways

Disadvantaged neighborhoods are known to predict adverse CVD outcomes [73]. Unger et al. [74] studied the association between neighborhood characteristics and cardiovascular health using baseline (2000–2002) data from the Multi-Ethnic Study of Atherosclerosis (MESA)—a national prospective cohort study nearly 7000 of middle aged and older adults in the US. The authors reported that resources for physical activity (OR 1.19; 95%CI 1.08–1.31), neighborhood walkability (OR 1.20; 95%CI 1.05–1.37) and high neighborhood SES (OR 1.20; 95%CI 1.05–1.37) were all associated with increased odds of ideal cardiovascular health score (cumulative measure of traditional CVD risk factors) [74].

The Jackson Heart Study—a landmark cohort study of over 4000 African American men and women aged 21–93 years—assessed the association between neighborhood disadvantage/poor social conditions and CVD risk, and found that each standard deviation (SD) increase in neighborhood disadvantage increased the risk of CVD by 25% (HR 1.25; 95% CI 1.05–1.49) in women but not in men [75]. The authors also reported an inverse relationship between neighborhood disadvantage, and duration/frequency of physical activity, with implications for overall CVD risk factor profile in disadvantaged communities. Similarly, findings from the Cardiovascular Health in Ambulatory Care Research Team (CANHEART) [76]—a large cross-sectional study of approximately 45,000 adults aged 40–70 years— showed a 19–33% higher 10-year CVD risk for individuals living in neighborhoods with low walkability scores, relative to residents of neighborhoods with high scores [76].

Other aspects of physical environment, such as air quality also have important effects on cardiovascular health. A systematic review of 18 studies (5 cohort and 13 cross-sectional) found that particulate matter air pollution was associated with the presence and progression of subclinical atherosclerosis, as measured by coronary artery calcium score and carotid intima media thickness [77]. Further, neighborhood safety might directly affect physical activity and possibly increase psychological stress—both risk factors for CVD [78, 79]. A cross-sectional study of the young and middle aged population in Stockholm, Sweden found that individuals living in unsafe neighborhoods with high crime rates experienced an up to 75% increased odds of CHD (OR 1.75; 95% CI 1.37–2.22) [78].

A cross-sectional study of 11,404 Australian adults reported a protective effect of neighborhood greenness (37% lower odds) on hospitalization for heart disease or stroke [80]. The Baltimore Memory Study, a cross-sectional study of 1,140 Baltimore residents aged 50–70 years, demonstrated that individuals in the most unsafe neighborhoods, as assessed by the self-reported neighborhood psychosocial hazards scale (NPH)—including indicators of public safety, physical disorder, economic deprivation and social disorganization—experienced over 4 times higher odds of myocardial infarction (MI) and 3 times higher odds of MI, stroke, transient ischemic attack (TIA), or intermittent claudication compared with residents living in safer neighborhoods [79].

Relatively little is known about the cumulative 'life course' effects of neighborhood disadvantage. While long-term effects of SES and neighborhood conditions have been examined overall, relatively few studies have examined such effects on cardiovascular outcomes [81–83]. Findings from a MESA study of nearly 5000 middle aged and older men and women, followed up for 20 years, suggest that worse neighborhood trajectory class (i.e. greater neighborhood poverty) predicted worse CVD outcomes, as measured by common carotid intima media thickness; however, the association was only observed in women. Greater research is needed to increase understanding of neighborhood and physical environment effects across the life course.

Summary

- *Neighborhood and physical environment provide, and facilitate access to, a variety of other SDOH*
- *Neighborhood environment affects CVD risk both directly as well as **via** behavioral and psychosocial pathways*
- *Weight of current evidence suggests a positive impact of favorable neighborhood conditions and a negative effect of unfavorable neighborhood conditions on overall cardiovascular health*
- *Further research is needed to better understand how exposure to adverse physical and psychosocial environments in early life predicts adverse CVD outcomes later in life*
- *Future efforts must examine the life-course perspective of disease and health in the context of neighborhoods, with particular attention to potential disparities in long-term outcomes by race/ethnicity*

Food

Dietary behaviors are an important part of traditional risk factor modification recommendations to promote cardiovascular health. Existing guidelines to reduce CVD risk via improvements in dietary habits have been extensively reviewed previously [84]. However, diet has mostly been analyzed in conjunction with other behavioral risk factors such as physical activity; much less attention has been paid to food as a distinct SDOH domain, particularly in the context of food insecurity—as discussed in this section.

Current Evidence and Pathways

Presence of nearby grocery stores and supermarkets is essential to availability of healthy food choices, which may improve overall cardiovascular risk profile. Kaiser et al. [85] used data from the MESA study to evaluate the relationship between neighborhood physical and social environment, and incident hypertension in nearly 3400 adults aged 45–84 years with a mean follow up of over 10 years; the authors reported that a 1 standard deviation (SD) increase in healthy food availability was associated with a 12% lower risk of hypertension (HR 0.88; 95%CI 0.82–0.95). Similarly, results from another MESA study of over 6800 US adults suggested that availability of 'favorable' food stores—defined as chain and non-chain supermarkets, and fruit and vegetable markets—was associated with 22% increased odds of a favorable cardiovascular profile (cumulative risk score based on traditional CVD risk factors) [74].

Morland et al. [86] studied the association between presence of supermarkets and convenience stores with CVD risk factors using data from over 10,000 adults enrolled in the ARIC study. The authors reported that prevalence of supermarkets was associated with lower prevalence of obesity (prevalence ratio [PR] 0.83; 95% CI 0.75–0.92) and overweight (PR 0.94; 95% CI 0.90–0.98); conversely, presence of convenience stores was associated with higher prevalence of both obesity (PR 1.16; 95% CI 1.05–1.27) and overweight (PR 1.06; 95% CI 1.02–1.10) [86]. Similar findings were documented by Powell and colleagues, who studied the association between access to local convenience stores vs supermarkets, and adolescent body mass index (BMI) in over 73,000 adolescents; [87] and reported that one additional chain supermarket per 10,000 capita was associated with 0.11 units lower BMI, and 0.6 percentage point reduction in overweight prevalence, whereas an additional convenience store per 10,000 capita was associated with 0.03 units higher BMI and 0.2 percentage points increase in prevalence of overweight [87].

Availability of healthy food choices may have important effects on CVD-related health behaviors. For example, Morland et al. [88] studied the contextual effects of local food environment on residents' diet using data from the ARIC study, and reported that presence of each additional supermarket in the census tract increased fruit and vegetable consumption by 32% and 11% in African Americans and Whites, respectively. However, low income neighborhoods are less likely to have healthy food outlets and supermarkets, and more likely to have small grocery and convenience stores [89]. Data from the 2000 Census [89] suggests considerable racial/ethnic and socioeconomic disparities in access to healthy food outlets, with 25% fewer chain supermarkets in low income neighborhoods, compared to middle-income neighborhoods; and 50–70% fewer chain supermarkets in African American and Hispanic neighborhoods, relative to White neighborhoods.

Living in a food desert—defined as area with both poor food access and low area income [90]—might increase risk of adverse CVD outcomes. A recent national cross-sectional study of nearly 9,000 young adults reported an increased cardiovascular health risk associated with residence in a food desert [91]. Similarly, a prospective study of nearly 5,000 middle aged and older individuals reported a 39% increased risk of MI and 18% increased risk of death from MI associated with living in a food desert, in patients with existing coronary artery disease (CAD); however, the association was observed only for low area income and not food access [92]. Greater research is needed to better understand the impact of environmental and contextual factors (e.g. nearby supermarkets) vs individual level barriers to access, such as income and/or other resources for accessing healthy food options (e.g. Supplemental Nutritional Assistance Program [SNAP] benefits, transportation, etc.).

Summary

- *Access to, and availability of healthy food is critical toward cardiovascular health, regardless of other sociodemographic determinants*
- *Both individual and area income, and availability of supermarkets and healthy food options are important from a primary and secondary CVD prevention perspective*
- *Further study is needed to better define—and measure—variables such as 'food access' that are often not well defined or appropriately analyzed in epidemiological studies*
- *Additional research is needed to understand the impact of economic resources (e.g. income, SNAP) on healthy food choices*
- *Public health programs should focus on developing evidence-based behavioral interventions that target enhanced utilization of healthy food options made available* via *supermarkets and grocery stores*
- *Community partnerships are key to improving access to healthy, affordable food*

Community and Social Context

Community and social context is defined as "the context in which societal and cultural factors interact to impact health outcomes" [93]. This domain is generally divided into four distinct sub-domains, including social support, social cohesion/social networks, community engagement and discrimination [3]. Each subdomain is subclassified to represent distinct constructs. For example, social support is often classified into the following four types: emotional, instrumental, informational and appraisal [94]. Similarly, discrimination is subdivided by (a) impact on specific population subgroups, such as racial/ethnic, national origin, gender, sexual orientation, elderly, and disabled; and (b) level of impact, such as individual and structural [3].

Current Evidence and Pathways

Each community and social context subdomain is linked to CVD via multiple, often interconnected pathways. For example, social support—a key subdomain—is linked to psychological wellbeing, increased ability to cope with stress, improved self-care and overall health-related quality of life [94, 95]. In a secondary analysis of randomized controlled trial (RCT) data from over 300 older adults with a history of heart failure (HF), Gallagher and colleagues found that individuals with high levels of social support were more likely to consult with a health professional for weight gain, adhere to medication, get a flu shot, and exercise regularly, compared to those with medium or low levels of social support [95].

Conversely, lack of social support has been associated with increased risk of CVD. In a secondary analysis of data for over 200 patients from two prospective studies, Wu et al. reported 2.5 times increased risk of adverse cardiac events in patients experiencing both lack of social support and medication non-adherence, relative to those with medication adherence and higher social support (OR) 2.47; 95% CI 1.16 5.23) [96]. In the same study, the authors reported a mediation effect of medication adherence on the social support-cardiac event-free survival relationship, highlighting a possible mechanism through which social support might impact cardiovascular health.

In one of the largest reported prospective cohort studies on the topic, Kawachi and colleagues [97] studied 32,624 male health professionals over a 4-year follow-up period, and reported that participants with the least social support had 1.9 times increased risk for cardiovascular mortality and 2.21 times increased risk of incident stroke, compared to those in the highest social support category (RR 1.90 & 2.21 for cardiovascular mortality and incident stroke, respectively).

While direct pathways from racism to CVD are relatively unclear, discrimination has been documented to have detrimental effects on overall cardiovascular health in marginalized populations [98]. A review of published empirical evidence (24 studies) of the link between racism/ethnic discrimination and hypertension found consistently elevated risk of hypertension in individuals experiencing racism; the observed patterns were more pronounced for institutional racism, compared to individual racism; and ambulatory blood pressure relative to resting blood pressure monitoring [99]. Similarly, results from the Metro Atlanta Heart Disease Study show that high psychological stress associated with racial discrimination is a strong predictor of incident hypertension in African Americans [100].

Social networks and social cohesion are important determinants of self-care and health. In a prospective study of 1,384 participants from the Cardiovascular and Metabolic Disease Etiology Research Center–High Risk Cohort, Joo and colleagues found that individuals with deficient social networks were 72% more likely to have higher CAC scores (>400) [101]. In addition, greater social cohesion has documented beneficial effects on cardiovascular health. For example, a prospective cohort study of over 500 middle aged and older women reported that each single point increase in social network index (SNI) score was associated with nearly 20% reduced risk of CVD mortality (Relative Risk [RR] 0.81; 95% CI 0.66–0.99); the authors reported that high SNI scores predicted lower total adverse cardiovascular events (combined mortality, hospitalization, MI, stroke, CHF; RR 0.85; 95% CI 0.75–0.96) and lower rehospitalization rates (RR 0.87; 95% CI 0.77–0.99) over the 2.3 year follow-up period [102].

The positive impacts of community engagement on cardiovascular health, and negative effects of a lack thereof, have been documented in the literature. In a unique cohort study of 2.8 million Swedish adults aged 45–74 years, low linking social capital (i.e. low community engagement) was associated with nearly 20% and 30% increased risk of CHD in men and women, respectively [103]. Conversely, in a convenience sample of middle aged and older African American women, Brown and colleagues demonstrated that a community engagement intervention for healthy behaviors was associated with improvements in cardiorespiratory fitness (Time to finish VO2max (min) = −1.87) and both systolic (−12.73 mmHg) and diastolic (−3.31 mmHg) blood pressure [104].

Summary

- *Existing evidence strongly suggests a negative effect of lack of/poor social support and social cohesion, and deficient social networks on cardiovascular health*
- *Evidence for a positive effect of social support—including the long-term impact of social support interventions—on CVD outcomes is less well documented in the literature*
- *Further evidence from large-scale, prospective studies is critical to clearly demonstrating the benefits of social support on cardiovascular health*
- *Greater quantitative and qualitative evidence is needed to develop a standardized social support measurement tool, with provisions for adaptation and use in a variety of sociodemographic settings*
- *Relatively few studies have examined the impact of race, racism and racial/ethnic discrimination on CVD; further study is warranted to elucidate potential mechanisms that explain the discrimination-CVD link in vulnerable populations*

Healthcare

Healthcare is a major SDOH. Given healthcare dynamics in the US, health insurance is a major determinant of access to essential health services; lack of which directly, and severely, limits access to health care and increases risk of adverse health outcomes, particularly among vulnerable and underserved minority population subgroups [105, 106].

Current Evidence and Pathways

It is known that being uninsured or underinsured diminishes the likelihood of receiving preventive care for CVD, increases the risk of missed doctor appointments and medication non-adherence, and is associated with poor overall cardiovascular health [107, 108]. A large-scale prospective study of over 15,000 middle aged and older adults reported that individuals without health insurance had 65% increased risk of stroke, and 26% increased risk of mortality, relative to the insured [109]. Further, the uninsured were less likely to be aware of CVD risk factors such as hypertension and hyperlipidemia, and less likely to report routine physical examination, compared to those with insurance coverage.

Disparities in access to care are a major driver of disparities in health outcomes, with a disproportionate impact on racial/ethnic minorities. Non-Hispanic Blacks and Hispanics make up the bulk of the uninsured population in the US, predisposing these already vulnerable populations to adverse CVD outcomes—as highlighted in multiple prior reports [29, 110–112]. Related, type of insurance is an important determinant of access to care. Findings from a nation-wide survey of 230,258 Medicaid beneficiaries indicated that this population is twice as likely to experience barriers to obtaining primary care, relative to those with private insurance [113]. For example, low re-imbursement for Medicaid patients has been cited as a possible reason for physicians not accepting Medicaid patients [114].

The beneficial effects of insurance coverage for the previously uninsured are well documented, [115] as evidenced by a household survey of 2203 middle aged and older adults, which showed that differences in CVD risk screening such as cholesterol screening between the insured and uninsured were reduced by nearly 20%, after the latter acquired Medicare coverage at the age of 65 [116]. Similarly, in a quasi-experimental study of over 1,000,000 US adults with CVD, Barghi et al. [117] reported positive outcomes with increased access to health services post ACA. The authors reported that, relative to the pre-ACA period (2012–2013), health insurance coverage, ability to pay for a doctor's visit and frequency of having an annual check-up increased by nearly 7, 3.6 and 2.2%, respectively in the post-ACA period (2015–2016).

In addition, transportation barriers, such as lack of access to personal vehicle or safe/reliable public transport may restrict access to, and utilization of health services, potentially resulting in delayed and/or missed care and prescription non-adherence [118].

A relatively under-investigated area is the issue of implicit provider bias in US healthcare, which might be based on race/ethnicity, SES, gender, weight and/or disability status. For example, findings from the Commonwealth Fund Minority Health Survey of US adult population document that low income is the most common reason for perceived discrimination [119]. In the same study, the authors reported that African Americans and Hispanics were more likely to report perceived discrimination, compared to White participants. Such biases affect patient-clinician interaction, medication adherence, treatment decisions, and overall quality of care and health outcomes [120].

Summary

- *Access, quality and timeliness of care are critical determinants of cardiovascular health*
- *Vulnerable population subgroups, including racial/ethnic minorities and the socioeconomically disadvantaged, face multiple health system barriers*
- *Lack of/limited insurance coverage, implicit bias and perceived discrimination predispose marginalized groups to higher CVD risk, and adverse CVD outcomes*
- *Major policy interventions are needed at local, state and federal levels to improve access to healthcare in minority populations*
- *Existing knowledge of the prevalence, and consequences of implicit bias and discrimination in healthcare is scant*
- *Future efforts must focus on studying, and addressing, both observed and implicit barriers to healthcare in underserved populations*

Conclusions

Disparities in CVD outcomes continue to affect vulnerable populations in the US adversely, and disproportionately. Existing disparities in both cardiovascular risk factors and major CVD outcomes cannot be reduced without effectively incorporating SDOH into CVD prevention and management paradigms. Recent social justice movements in the US have attracted much needed attention toward inequities in healthcare; however, SDOH remain grossly underutilized in contemporary clinical practice models, to the detriment of the individual patient and the healthcare system.

Policy initiatives to improve individual and population level health outcomes, reduce health inequities, and provide evidence-based personalized care, such as the Precision Medicine Initiative (2015) [14] and 21st Century Cures Act (2016), [15] hinge on integrative care models that must effectively incorporate individuals' unique SDOH burden. Recent efforts to achieve these goals, such as The National Association of Community Health Center's (NACHC) Protocol for Responding to and Assessing Patients' Assets, Risks, and Experiences (PRAPARE)

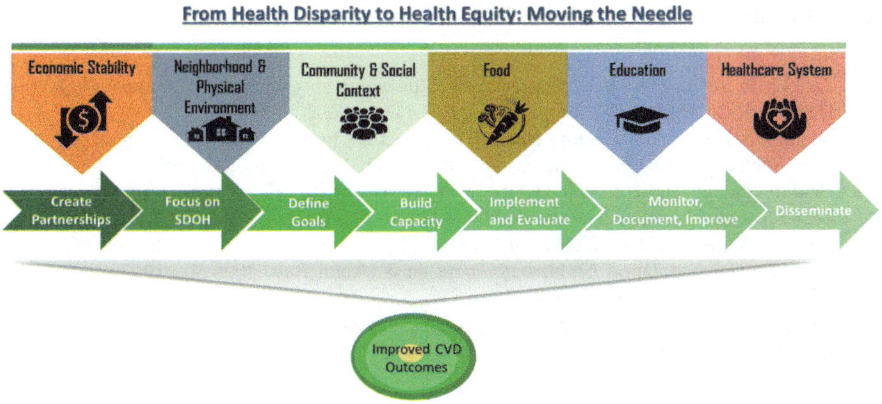

Fig. 2 On the road to health equity

Implementation and Action Toolkit offer great promise, and exciting opportunities for future work in the field [121]. Future efforts must focus on development and validation of these and similar tools in a variety of clinical settings, including CVD.

Meaningful synthesis, use and application of SDOH knowledge to design equitable care models, and narrow CVD disparities will require rigorous and coordinated efforts on the following fronts (Fig. 2):

1. Large-scale efforts to collect data on SDOH in local, regional and national data streams, including surveys, registries and clinical/claims databases.
2. Ensure accuracy of race/ethnicity data to generate reliable estimates of racial/ethnic disparities in cardiovascular outcomes in the US.
3. Greater use of existing population health databases to examine both cross-sectional and longitudinal effects of SDOH on CVD risk factors and outcomes.
4. Use knowledge generated from item 3 to design and implement evidence-based public health interventions, targeting 'upstream' and 'midstream' factors.
5. Train the new generation of healthcare workforce to understand the burden and implications of health disparities in the US; include modules on cultural competence and implicit bias in medical school and residency training curricula.
6. Create multidisciplinary teams of clinicians, data scientists and population health experts in order to harmonize efforts to achieve health equity.

References

1. Zabel MR, Stevens DP. What happens to health care quality when the patient pays? Qual Saf Heal Care. 2006;15:146–7. https://doi.org/10.1136/qshc.2006.018531.
2. Social Determinants of Health | Healthy People 2020. https://www.healthypeople.gov/2020/topics-objectives/topic/social-determinants-of-health. Accessed 5 Nov 2020.
3. Healthy People 2030. Social Determinants of Health. Retrieved from https://health.gov/healthypeople/objectives-and-data/social-determinants-health.
4. Harvey PW. Social determinants of health—why we continue to ignore them in the search for improved population health outcomes! Aust Health Rev. 2006;30:419–23. https://doi.org/10.1071/AH060419.
5. Benjamin RM. Surgeon general's perspectives: the national prevention strategy: shifting the nation's health-care system. Public Health Rep. 2011;126:774–6. https://doi.org/10.1177/003335491112600602.
6. Vilhelmsson A. Value-based health care delivery, preventive medicine and the medicalization of public health. cureus 2017;9. https://doi.org/10.7759/cureus.1063.
7. Levine S, Malone E, Lekiachvili A, Briss P. Health care industry insights: why the use of preventive services is still low. Prev Chronic Dis. 2019;16. https://doi.org/10.5888/pcd16.180625.
8. Social Determinants of Health (SDOH). https://catalyst.nejm.org/doi/full/10.1056/CAT.17.0312. Accessed 7 Dec 2020.
9. Parikh RB, Jain SH, Navathe AS. The sociobehavioral phenotype: applying a precision medicine framework to social determinants of health. Am J Manag Care. 2019;25. https://pubmed.ncbi.nlm.nih.gov/31518090/. Accessed 7 Dec 2020.
10. Hekler E, Tiro JA, Hunter CM, Nebeker C. Precision health: the role of the social and behavioral sciences in advancing the vision. Ann Behav Med. 2020;54:805–26. https://doi.org/10.1093/abm/kaaa018.
11. American Academy of Family Physicians. Addressing Social Determinants of Health in Primary Care. https://www.aafp.org/dam/AAFP/documents/patient_care/everyone_project/team-based-approach.pdf 2018.
12. McGrath SP. Improving the Odds of success for precision medicine using the social ecological model. AMIA Annu Symp Proceedings AMIA Symp. 2019;2019:1149–56.
13. Olstad DL, McIntyre L. Reconceptualising precision public health. BMJ Open 2019;9. https://doi.org/https://doi.org/10.1136/bmjopen-2019-030279.
14. Duffy DJ. Problems, challenges and promises: perspectives on precision medicine. Brief Bioinform. 2016;17:494–504. https://doi.org/10.1093/bib/bbv060.
15. Glasgow RE, Kwan BM, Matlock DD. Realizing the full potential of precision health: The need to include patient-reported health behavior, mental health, social determinants, and patient preferences data. J Clin Transl Sci. 2018;2:183–5. https://doi.org/10.1017/cts.2018.31.
16. Peikes D, Chen A, Schore J, Brown R. Effects of care coordination on hospitalization, quality of care, and health care expenditures among medicare beneficiaries 15 randomized trials. JAMA—J Am Med Assoc. 2009;301:603–18. https://doi.org/10.1001/jama.2009.126.
17. O'Toole TP, Johnson EE, Aiello R, Kane V, Pape L. Tailoring care to vulnerable populations by incorporating social determinants of health: the veterans health administration's "homeless patient aligned care team" program. Prev Chronic Dis. 2016;13. https://doi.org/10.5888/pcd13.150567.
18. Bradley EH, Canavan M, Rogan E, Talbert-Slagle K, Ndumele C, Taylor L, et al. Variation in health outcomes: the role of spending on social services, public health, and health care, 2000–09. Health Aff. 2016;35:760–8. https://doi.org/10.1377/hlthaff.2015.0814.
19. National Minority Health Month. n.d. https://minorityhealth.hhs.gov/heckler30/. Accessed 5 Nov 2020.

20. Smedley BD, Stith AY, Nelson AR. Unequal treatment: confronting racial and ethnic disparities in health care (with CD). National Academies Press; 2003. https://doi.org/https://doi.org/10.17226/12875.

21. Racial/Ethnic Differences in Cardiac Care: The Weight of the Evidence | KFF. n.d. https://www.kff.org/racial-equity-and-health-policy/fact-sheet/racialethnic-differences-in-cardiac-care-the-weight/. Accessed 5 November 2020.

22. CDC Health Disparities & Inequalities Report (CHDIR)—Minority Health—CDC. 2013. https://www.cdc.gov/minorityhealth/CHDIReport.html. Accessed 5 Nov 2020.

23. White-Williams C, Rossi LP, Bittner VA, Driscoll A, Durant RW, Granger BB, et al. Addressing social determinants of health in the care of patients with heart failure: a scientific statement from the american heart association. Circulation. 2020;141:E841–63. https://doi.org/10.1161/CIR.0000000000000767.

24. Havranek EP, Mujahid MS, Barr DA, Blair IV, Cohen MS, Cruz-Flores S, et al. Social determinants of risk and outcomes for cardiovascular disease: a scientific statement from the American heart association. Circulation. 2015;132:873–98. https://doi.org/10.1161/CIR.0000000000000228.

25. Benjamin EJ, Muntner P, Alonso A, Bittencourt MS, Callaway CW, Carson AP, et al. Heart disease and stroke statistics-2019 update: a report from the american heart association. Circulation. 2019;139:e56-528. https://doi.org/10.1161/CIR.0000000000000659.

26. Nelson S, Whitsel L, Khavjou O, Phelps D, Leib A. Projections of cardiovascular disease prevalence and costs. American Heart Association. 2016. https://www.heart.org/idc/groups/heart-public/@wcm/@adv/documents/downloadable/ucm_491513.pdf.

27. Center for Health Statistics. Racial and Ethnic Disparities in Heart Disease. 2019. https://www.cdc.gov/nchs/hus/spotlight/HeartDiseaseSpotlight_2019_0404.pdf.

28. Youmans QR, Hastings-Spaine L, Princewill O, Shobayo T, Okwuosa IS. Disparities in cardiovascular care: past, present, and solutions. Cleve Clin J Med. 2019;86:621–32. https://doi.org/10.3949/ccjm.86a.18088.

29. FACTS: Bridging the Gap CVD Health Disparities. 2012. American Heart Association. https://www.heart.org/idc/groups/heart-public/@wcm/@adv/documents/downloadable/ucm_301731.pdf.

30. Abstract 19538: Racial Disparities in the Utilization of Cardiovascular Disease Preventive Care Services in the United States: Insight From Medical Expenditure Panel Survey 2014 | Circulation. n.d. https://www.ahajournals.org/doi/https://doi.org/10.1161/circ.136.suppl_1.19538. Accessed 16 Nov 2020.

31. Abdalla SM, Yu S, Galea S. Trends in Cardiovascular disease prevalence by income level in the United States. JAMA Netw Open. 2020;3. https://doi.org/10.1001/jamanetworkopen.2020.18150.

32. Braveman P, Gottlieb L. The social determinants of health: It's time to consider the causes of the causes. Public Health Rep. 2014;129:19–31. https://doi.org/10.1177/00333549141291s206.

33. Gehlert S, Sohmer D, Sacks T, Mininger C, McClintock M, Olopade O. Targeting health disparities: a model linking upstream determinants to downstream interventions. Health Aff. 2008;27:339–49. https://doi.org/10.1377/hlthaff.27.2.339.

34. Kaplan GA. Social determinants of health, 2nd Edition. M Marmot, R Wilkinson (eds). Oxford: Oxford University Press, 2006, pp. 376, $57.50. ISBN: 9780198565895. Int J Epidemiol. 2006;35:1111–2. https://doi.org/https://doi.org/10.1093/ije/dyl121.

35. Kreatsoulas C, Anand SS. The impact of social determinants on cardiovascular disease. Can J Cardiol. vol. 26, Pulsus Group Inc.; 2010, p. 8C–13C. https://doi.org/https://doi.org/10.1016/S0828-282X(10)71075-8.

36. Hood CM, Gennuso KP, Swain GR, Catlin BB. County health rankings: relationships between determinant factors and health outcomes. Am J Prev Med. 2016;50:129–35. https://doi.org/10.1016/j.amepre.2015.08.024.

37. Social Determinants of Health—Healthy People 2030 | health.gov. n.d. https://health.gov/healthypeople/objectives-and-data/social-determinants-health. Accessed 5 Nov 2020.

38. Magnan S. Social determinants of health 101 for health care: Five Plus Five. NAM Perspect 2017;7. https://doi.org/https://doi.org/10.31478/201710c.

39. Kivimäki M, Shipley MJ, Ferrie JE, Singh-Manoux A, Batty GD, Chandola T, et al. Best-practice interventions to reduce socioeconomic inequalities of coronary heart disease mortality in UK: a prospective occupational cohort study. Lancet. 2008;372:1648–54. https://doi.org/10.1016/S0140-6736(08)61688-8.

40. Chow CK, Lock K, Teo K, Subramanian S, McKee M, Yusuf S. Environmental and societal influences acting on cardiovascular risk factors and disease at a population level: a review. Int J Epidemiol. 2009;38:1580–94. https://doi.org/10.1093/ije/dyn258.

41. Mensah GA, Mokdad AH, Ford ES, Greenlund KJ, Croft JB. State of disparities in cardiovascular health in the United States. Circulation, vol. 111, Lippincott Williams & Wilkins; 2005, p. 1233–41. https://doi.org/https://doi.org/10.1161/01.CIR.0000158136. 76824.04.

42. Beyond Health Care: The Role of Social Determinants in Promoting Health and Health Equity | KFF. n.d. https://www.kff.org/racial-equity-and-health-policy/issue-brief/beyond-health-care-the-role-of-social-determinants-in-promoting-health-and-health-equity/. Accessed 5 Nov 2020.

43. Fretz A, Schneider ALC, McEvoy JW, Hoogeveen R, Ballantyne CM, Coresh J, et al. The association of socioeconomic status with subclinical myocardial damage, incident cardiovascular events, and mortality in the ARIC study. Am J Epidemiol. 2016;183:452–61. https://doi.org/10.1093/aje/kwv253.

44. Marshall IJ, Wang Y, Crichton S, McKevitt C, Rudd AG, Wolfe CDA. The effects of socioeconomic status on stroke risk and outcomes. Lancet Neurol. 2015;14:1206–18. https://doi.org/10.1016/S1474-4422(15)00200-8.

45. Hamad R, Penko J, Kazi DS, Coxson P, Guzman D, Wei PC, et al. Association of low socioeconomic status with premature coronary heart disease in US adults. JAMA Cardiol. 2020;5. https://doi.org/https://doi.org/10.1001/jamacardio.2020.1458.

46. Manrique-Garcia E, Sidorchuk A, Hallqvist J, Moradi T. Socioeconomic position and incidence of acute myocardial infarction: a meta-analysis. J Epidemiol Community Health. 2011;65:301–9. https://doi.org/10.1136/jech.2009.104075.

47. Leng B, Jin Y, Li G, Chen L, Jin N. Socioeconomic status and hypertension. J Hypertens. 2015;33:221–9. https://doi.org/10.1097/HJH.0000000000000428.

48. Marmot MG, Shipley MJ, Rose G. Inequalities in death-specific explanations of a general pattern? Lancet. 1984;323:1003–6. https://doi.org/10.1016/S0140-6736(84)92337-7.

49. Addo J, Ayerbe L, Mohan KM, Crichton S, Sheldenkar A, Chen R, et al. Socioeconomic status and stroke: an updated review. Stroke. 2012;43:1186–91. https://doi.org/10.1161/STROKEAHA.111.639732.

50. Stirbu I, Looman C, Nijhof GJ, Reulings PG, Mackenbach JP. Income inequalities in case death of ischaemic heart disease in the Netherlands: a national record-linked study. n.d. https://doi.org/https://doi.org/10.1136/jech-2011-200924.

51. Wang SY, Tan ASL, Claggett B, Chandra A, Khatana SAM, Lutsey PL, et al. Longitudinal associations between income changes and incident cardiovascular disease: the atherosclerosis risk in communities study. JAMA Cardiol. 2019;4:1203–12. https://doi.org/10.1001/jamacardio.2019.3788.

52. Eshak ES, Honjo K, Iso H, Ikeda A, Inoue M, Sawada N, et al. Changes in the employment status and risk of stroke and stroke types. Stroke. 2017;48:1176–82. https://doi.org/10.1161/STROKEAHA.117.016967.

53. Mellis AM, Athamneh LN, Stein JS, Sze YY, Epstein LH, Bickel WK. Less is more: negative income shock increases immediate preference in cross commodity discounting and food demand. Appetite. 2018;129:155–61. https://doi.org/10.1016/j.appet.2018.06.032.

54. Lett HS, Blumenthal JA, Babyak MA, Sherwoob A, Strauman T, Robins C, et al. Depression as a risk factor for coronary artery disease: evidence, mechanisms, and treatment. Psychosom Med. 2004;66:305–15. https://doi.org/10.1097/01.psy.0000126207.43307.c0.

55. Holahan J. The 2007–09 recession and health insurance coverage. Health Aff. 2011;30:145–52. https://doi.org/10.1377/hlthaff.2010.1003.
56. Social conditions as fundamental causes of disease—PubMed. n.d. https://pubmed.ncbi.nlm.nih.gov/7560851/. Accessed 5 Nov 2020.
57. Skevington SM. Qualities of life, educational level and human development: an international investigation of health. Soc Psychiatry Psychiatr Epidemiol. 2010;45:999–1009. https://doi.org/10.1007/s00127-009-0138-x.
58. Khaing W, Vallibhakara SA, Attia J, McEvoy M, Thakkinstian A. Effects of education and income on cardiovascular outcomes: A systematic review and meta-analysis. Eur J Prev Cardiol. 2017;24:1032–42. https://doi.org/10.1177/2047487317705916.
59. Rosengren A, Smyth A, Rangarajan S, Ramasundarahettige C, Bangdiwala SI, AlHabib KF, et al. Socioeconomic status and risk of cardiovascular disease in 20 low-income, middle-income, and high-income countries: the Prospective Urban Rural Epidemiologic (PURE) study. Lancet Glob Heal. 2019;7:e748–60. https://doi.org/10.1016/S2214-109X(19)30045-2.
60. Rosengren A, Subramanian S V, Islam S, Chow CK, Avezum A, Kazmi K, et al. Education and risk for acute myocardial infarction in 52 high, middle and low-income countries: INTERHEART case-control study. n.d. https://doi.org/https://doi.org/10.1136/hrt.2009.182436.
61. Kubota Y, Heiss G, Maclehose RF, Roetker NS, Folsom AR. Association of educational attainment with lifetime risk of cardiovascular disease the atherosclerosis risk in communities study. JAMA Intern Med. 2017;177:1165–72. https://doi.org/10.1001/jamainternmed.2017.1877.
62. Measuring the value of education: Career Outlook: U.S. Bureau of Labor Statistics. n.d. https://www.bls.gov/careeroutlook/2018/data-on-display/education-pays.htm. Accessed 5 Nov 2020.
63. Zajacova A, Lawrence EM. The relationship between education and health: reducing disparities through a contextual approach. Annu Rev Public Heal. 2018;39:273–89. https://doi.org/10.1146/annurev-publhealth.
64. Institute U, Dubay L, Simon SM, Zimmerman E, Luk KX, Woolf SH. How are income and wealth linked to health and longevity? laudan aron Center on Society and Health. 2015.
65. Loucks EB, Pilote L, Lynch JW, Richard H, Almeida ND, Benjamin EJ, et al. Life course socioeconomic position is associated with inflammatory markers: the framingham offspring study. Soc Sci Med. 2010;71:187–95. https://doi.org/10.1016/j.socscimed.2010.03.012.
66. Berkman ND, Sheridan SL, Donahue KE, Halpern DJ, Crotty K. Low health literacy and health outcomes: an updated systematic review. Ann Intern Med. 2011;155:97–107. https://doi.org/10.7326/0003-4819-155-2-201107190-00005.
67. Phelan JC, Link BG, Tehranifar P. Social conditions as fundamental causes of health inequalities: theory, evidence, and policy implications. J Health Soc Behav. 2010;51:S28-40. https://doi.org/10.1177/0022146510383498.
68. Ahluwalia JS, Richter K, Mayo MS, Ahluwalia HK, Choi WS, Schmelzle KH, et al. African American smokers interested and eligible for a smoking cessation clinical trial: predictors of not returning for randomization. Ann Epidemiol. 2002;12:206–12. https://doi.org/10.1016/S1047-2797(01)00305-2.
69. Youmans SL, Schillinger D. Functional health literacy and medication use: the pharmacist's role. Ann Pharmacother. 2003;37:1726–9. https://doi.org/10.1345/aph.1D070.
70. Kelli HM, Mehta A, Tahhan AS, Liu C, Kim JH, Dong TA, et al. Low educational attainment is a predictor of adverse outcomes in patients with coronary artery disease. J Am Heart Assoc. 2019;8. https://doi.org/10.1161/JAHA.119.013165.
71. Kalichman SC, Ramachandran B, Catz S. Adherence to combination antiretroviral therapies in HIV patients of low health literacy. J Gen Intern Med. 1999;14:267–73. https://doi.org/10.1046/j.1525-1497.1999.00334.x.

72. DeWalt DA, Berkman ND, Sheridan S, Lohr KN, Pignone MP. Literacy and health outcomes: a systematic review of the literature. J Gen Intern Med. 2004;19:1228–39. https://doi.org/10.1111/j.1525-1497.2004.40153.x.

73. Koohsari MJ, McCormack GR, Nakaya T, Oka K. Neighbourhood built environment and cardiovascular disease: knowledge and future directions. Nat Rev Cardiol. 2020;17:261–3. https://doi.org/10.1038/s41569-020-0343-6.

74. Unger E, Diez-Roux AV, Lloyd-Jones DM, Mujahid MS, Nettleton JA, Bertoni A, et al. Association of neighborhood characteristics with cardiovascular health in the multi-ethnic study of atherosclerosis. Circ Cardiovasc Qual Outcomes. 2014;7:524–31. https://doi.org/10.1161/CIRCOUTCOMES.113.000698.

75. Barber S, Hickson DA, Wang X, Sims M, Nelson C, Diez-Roux AV. Neighborhood disadvantage, poor social conditions, and cardiovascular disease incidence among African American adults in the Jackson heart study. Am J Public Health. 2016;106:2219–26. https://doi.org/10.2105/AJPH.2016.303471.

76. Howell NA, Tu J V., Moineddin R, Chu A, Booth GL. Association between neighborhood walkability and predicted 10-year cardiovascular disease risk: the CANHEART (Cardiovascular Health in Ambulatory Care Research Team) cohort. J Am Heart Assoc. 2019;8. https://doi.org/https://doi.org/10.1161/JAHA.119.013146.

77. Jilani MH, Simon-Friedt B, Yahya T, Khan AY, Hassan SZ, Kash B, et al. Associations between particulate matter air pollution, presence and progression of subclinical coronary and carotid atherosclerosis: a systematic review. Atherosclerosis. 2020;306:22–32. https://doi.org/10.1016/j.atherosclerosis.2020.06.018.

78. Sundquist K, Theobald H, Yang M, Li X, Johansson SE, Sundquist J. Neighborhood violent crime and unemployment increase the risk of coronary heart disease: a multilevel study in an urban setting. Soc Sci Med. 2006;62:2061–71. https://doi.org/10.1016/j.socscimed.2005.08.051.

79. Augustin T, Glass TA, James BD, Schwartz BS. Neighborhood psychosocial hazards and cardiovascular disease: the baltimore memory study. Am J Public Health. 2008;98:1664–70. https://doi.org/10.2105/AJPH.2007.125138.

80. Pereira G, Foster S, Martin K, Christian H, Boruff BJ, Knuiman M, et al. The association between neighborhood greenness and cardiovascular disease: an observational study. BMC Public Health. 2012;12:466. https://doi.org/10.1186/1471-2458-12-466.

81. Jivraj S, Murray ET, Norman P, Nicholas O. The impact of life course exposures to neighbourhood deprivation on health and well-being: a review of the long-term neighbourhood effects literature. Eur J Public Health. 2020;30:922–8. https://doi.org/10.1093/eurpub/ckz153.

82. Clarke P, Morenoff J, Debbink M, Golberstein E, Elliott MR, Lantz PM. Cumulative exposure to neighborhood context: consequences for health transitions over the adult life course. Res Aging. 2014;36:115–42. https://doi.org/10.1177/0164027512470702.

83. Murray ET, Diez Roux AV, Carnethon M, Lutsey PL, Ni H, O'Meara ES. Trajectories of neighborhood poverty and associations with subclinical atherosclerosis and associated risk factors. Am J Epidemiol. 2010;171:1099–108. https://doi.org/10.1093/aje/kwq044.

84. Krauss RM, Eckel RH, Howard B, Appel LJ, Daniels SR, Deckelbaum RJ, et al. AHA dietary guidelines. Circulation. 2000;102:2284–99. https://doi.org/10.1161/01.CIR.102.18.2284.

85. Kaiser P, Diez Roux A V., Mujahid M, Carnethon M, Bertoni A, Adar SD, et al. Neighborhood environments and incident hypertension in the multi-ethnic study of atherosclerosis. Am J Epidemiol., vol. 183, Oxford University Press; 2016, p. 988–97. https://doi.org/https://doi.org/10.1093/aje/kwv296.

86. Morland K, Diez Roux AV, Wing S. Supermarkets, other food stores, and obesity: the atherosclerosis risk in communities study. Am J Prev Med. 2006;30:333–9. https://doi.org/10.1016/j.amepre.2005.11.003.

87. Powell LM, Auld MC, Chaloupka FJ, O'Malley PM, Johnston LD. Associations between access to food stores and adolescent body mass index. Am J Prev Med. 2007;33:S301–7. https://doi.org/10.1016/j.amepre.2007.07.007.

88. Morland K, Wing S, Roux AD. The contextual effect of the local food environment on residents' diets: The atherosclerosis risk in communities study. Am J Public Health. 2002;92:1761–7. https://doi.org/10.2105/ajph.92.11.1761.

89. Powell LM, Slater S, Mirtcheva D, Bao Y, Chaloupka FJ. Food store availability and neighborhood characteristics in the United States. Prev Med (Baltim). 2007;44:189–95. https://doi.org/10.1016/j.ypmed.2006.08.008.

90. USDA ERS—Documentation. 2020. https://www.ers.usda.gov/data-products/food-access-research-atlas/documentation/. Accessed 17 Nov 2020.

91. Testa A, Jackson DB, Semenza DC, Vaughn MG. Food deserts and cardiovascular health among young adults. Public Health Nutr 2020:1–8. https://doi.org/https://doi.org/10.1017/S1368980020001536.

92. Kelli HM, Kim JH, Tahhan AS, Liu C, Ko YA, Hammadah M, et al. Living in food deserts and adverse cardiovascular outcomes in patients with cardiovascular disease. J Am Heart Assoc 2019;8. https://doi.org/https://doi.org/10.1161/JAHA.118.010694.

93. Hernandez LM, Blazer DG. Genes, behavior, and the social environment: moving beyond the nature/nurture debate. National Academies Press; 2006. https://doi.org/https://doi.org/10.17226/11693.

94. Langford CPH, Bowsher J, Maloney JP, Lillis PP. Social support: a conceptual analysis. J Adv Nurs. 1997;25:95–100. https://doi.org/https://doi.org/10.1046/j.1365-2648.1997.1997025095.x.

95. Gallagher R, Luttik M-L, Jaarsma T. Social support and self-care in heart failure. J Cardiovasc Nurs. 2011;26:439–45. https://doi.org/10.1097/JCN.0b013e31820984e1.

96. Wu JR, Frazier SK, Rayens MK, Lennie TA, Chung ML, Moser DK. Medication adherence, social support, and event-free survival in patients with heart failure. Heal Psychol. 2013;32:637–46. https://doi.org/10.1037/a0028527.

97. Kawachi I, Colditz GA, Ascherio A, Rimm EB, Giovannucci E, Stampfer MJ, et al. A prospective study of social networks in relation to total mortality and cardiovascular disease in men in the USA. J Epidemiol Community Health. 1996;50:245–51. https://doi.org/10.1136/jech.50.3.245.

98. Cozier Y, Palmer JR, Horton NJ, Fredman L, Wise LA, Rosenberg L. Racial Discrimination and the Incidence of Hypertension in US Black Women. Ann Epidemiol. 2006;16:681–7. https://doi.org/10.1016/j.annepidem.2005.11.008.

99. Brondolo E, Love EE, Pencille M, Schoenthaler A, Ogedegbe G. Racism and hypertension: a review of the empirical evidence and implications for clinical practice. Am J Hypertens. 2011;24:518–29. https://doi.org/10.1038/ajh.2011.9.

100. Stress-related racial discrimination and hypertension likelihood in a population-based sample of African Americans: the Metro Atlanta Heart Disease Study—PubMed. n.d. https://pubmed.ncbi.nlm.nih.gov/16259480/. Accessed 6 Nov 2020.

101. Joo WT, Lee CJ, Oh J, Kim IC, Lee SH, Kang SM, et al. The association between social network betweenness and coronary calcium: A baseline study of patients with a high risk of cardiovascular disease. J Atheroscler Thromb. 2018;25:131–41. https://doi.org/10.5551/jat.40469.

102. Rutledge T, Reis SE, Olson M, Owens J, Kelsey SF, Pepine CJ, et al. Social networks are associated with lower mortality rates among women with suspected coronary disease: The national heart, lung, and blood institute-sponsored women's ischemia syndrome evaluation study. Psychosom Med. 2004;66:882–8. https://doi.org/10.1097/01.psy.0000145819.94041.52.

103. Sundquist J, Johansson SE, Yang M, Sundquist K. Low linking social capital as a predictor of coronary heart disease in Sweden: a cohort study of 2.8 million people. Soc Sci Med. 2006;62:954–63. https://doi.org/https://doi.org/10.1016/j.socscimed.2005.06.049.

104. Brown AGM, Hudson LB, Chui K, Metayer N, Lebron-Torres N, Seguin RA, et al. Improving heart health among Black/African American women using civic engagement: a pilot study. BMC Public Health. 2017;17:112. https://doi.org/10.1186/s12889-016-3964-2.
105. IOM. Unequal Treatment: Confronting Racial and Ethnic Disparities in Health Care : Health and Medicine Division. 2002. https://www.nationalacademies.org/hmd/Reports/2002/Unequal-Treatment-Confronting-Racial-and-Ethnic-Disparities-in-Health-Care.aspx. Accessed 6 Nov 2019.
106. Call KT, McAlpine DD, Garcia CM, Shippee N, Beebe T, Adeniyi TC, et al. Barriers to care in an ethnically diverse publicly insured population: Is health care reform enough? Med Care. 2014;52:720–7. https://doi.org/10.1097/MLR.0000000000000172.
107. America's uninsured crisis: Consequences for health and health care. National Academies Press; 2009. https://doi.org/https://doi.org/10.17226/12511.
108. Khera R, Valero-Elizondo J, Das SR, Virani SS, Kash BA, De Lemos JA, et al. Cost-related medication nonadherence in adults with atherosclerotic cardiovascular disease in the United States, 2013 to 2017. Circulation. 2019;140:2067–75. https://doi.org/10.1161/CIRCULATIONAHA.119.041974.
109. Fowler-Brown A, Corbie-Smith G, Garrett J, Lurie N. Risk of cardiovascular events and death - does insurance matter? J Gen Intern Med. 2007;22:502–7. https://doi.org/10.1007/s11606-007-0127-2.
110. The Uninsured and the ACA: A Primer—Key Facts about Health Insurance and the Uninsured amidst Changes to the Affordable Care Act | KFF n.d. https://www.kff.org/uninsured/report/the-uninsured-and-the-aca-a-primer-key-facts-about-health-insurance-and-the-uninsured-amidst-changes-to-the-affordable-care-act/. Accessed 6 Nov 2020.
111. Adam Leigh J, Alvarez M, Rodriguez CJ. Ethnic minorities and coronary heart disease: An update and future directions. Curr Atheroscler Rep. 2016;18:9. https://doi.org/10.1007/s11883-016-0559-4.
112. Muncan B. Cardiovascular disease in racial/ethnic minority populations: Illness burden and overview of community-based interventions 11 Medical and Health Sciences 1102 Cardiorespiratory Medicine and Haematology 11 Medical and Health Sciences 1117 Public Health and Health Services Henrique Barros, Bent Greve. Walter Ricciardi Public Health Rev. 2018;39:32. https://doi.org/10.1186/s40985-018-0109-4.
113. Cheung PT, Wiler JL, Lowe RA, Ginde AA. National study of barriers to timely primary care and emergency department utilization among medicaid beneficiaries. Ann Emerg Med. 2012;60(4–10). https://doi.org/10.1016/j.annemergmed.2012.01.035.
114. Cunningham P, May J. Medicaid patients increasingly concentrated among physicians. Tracking Report. 2006. https://pubmed.ncbi.nlm.nih.gov/16918046/.
115. Buchmueller TC, Grumbach K, Kronick R, Kahn JG. The effect of health insurance on medical care utilization and implications for insurance expansion: a review of the literature. Med Care Res Rev. 2005;62:3–30. https://doi.org/10.1177/1077558704271718.
116. McWilliams JM, Zaslavsky AM, Meara E, Ayanian JZ. Impact of medicare coverage on basic clinical services for previously uninsured adults. J Am Med Assoc. 2003;290:757–64. https://doi.org/10.1001/jama.290.6.757.
117. Barghi A, Torres H, Kressin NR, McCormick D. Coverage and access for Americans with cardiovascular disease or risk factors after the ACA: a quasi-experimental Study. J Gen Intern Med. 2019;34:1797–805. https://doi.org/10.1007/s11606-019-05108-1.
118. Syed ST, Gerber BS, Sharp LK. Traveling towards disease: transportation barriers to health care access. J Community Health. 2013;38:976–93. https://doi.org/10.1007/s10900-013-9681-1.
119. LaVeist TA, Rolley NC, Diala C. Prevalence and patterns of discrimination among U.S. health care consumers. Int J Heal Serv. 2003;33:331–44. https://doi.org/https://doi.org/10.2190/TCAC-P90F-ATM5-B5U0.

120. Hall WJ, Chapman MV, Lee KM, Merino YM, Thomas TW, Payne BK, et al. Implicit racial/ethnic bias among health care professionals and its influence on health care outcomes: a systematic review. Am J Public Health. 2015;105:e60-76. https://doi.org/10.2105/AJPH. 2015.302903.
121. PRAPARE Implementation and Action Toolkit. 2019. https://www.nachc.org/research-and-data/prapare/toolkit/. Accessed 7 Dec 2020.
122. Kilander L, Berglund L, Boberg M, Vessby B, Lithell H. Education, lifestyle factors and mortality fromcardiovascular disease and cancer. A 25-year follow-up of Swedish 50-year-old men. Int J Epidemiol 2001;30(5):1119–1126. https://doi.org/10.1093/ije/30.5. 1119

Biomarkers

Renato Quispe, Thomas Das, and Erin D. Michos

Introduction

Due to the heterogenous and multifactorial nature of cardiovascular disease (CVD), it can be difficult to predict which asymptomatic individuals are at increased risk for developing symptomatic disease. Matching the intensity of treatment with the absolute risk of the patient is the core tenet of precision medicine. Following a healthy lifestyle throughout one's lifespan is the foundation for CVD prevention. For those determined to be at elevated risk for an atherosclerotic CVD (ASCVD) event, HMG-CoA reductase inhibitors (statins) are first line pharmacotherapy for reducing ASCVD risk across all major guidelines [1–3]. However, risk estimation tools based on traditional CVD risk factors, such as the Pooled Cohort Equations (PCE), which are derived from population averages, are imprecise for a given individual [4–6]. This entire book is devoted to genetic, imaging, and other strategies to improve precision in CVD risk estimation, and this chapter will focus on the role of biomarkers.

Biomarkers, which are often used in conjunction with traditional risk factors, are subclinical indicators of physiological and pathological processes [7]. Biomarkers can serve as useful tools in facilitating prognostication of CVD risk and disease progression [8], as well as assessment of cardiovascular health [9]. Elevation of cardiac biomarkers can help identify the individuals at increased risk of incidence and progression of disease who may benefit from more intensive medical therapy. Compared to imaging-based risk markers such as coronary artery calcium (CAC),

R. Quispe · T. Das
The Ciccarone Center for Cardiovascular Disease Prevention, Johns Hopkins University School of Medicine, Baltimore, MD, USA

E. D. Michos (✉)
Ciccarone Center for the Prevention of Cardiovascular Disease, Johns Hopkins Hospital, 600 N. Wolfe Street, Blalock 524-B, Baltimore, MD 21287, USA
e-mail: edonnell@jhmi.edu

© Springer Nature Switzerland AG 2021

31

S. S. Martin (ed.), *Precision Medicine in Cardiovascular Disease Prevention*,
https://doi.org/10.1007/978-3-030-75055-8_2

measurement of biomarkers has the advantage of no radiation exposure and can easily be done from a single blood draw, often alongside other clinical laboratory measures. Clinically useful biomarkers are molecules that can be repeatedly and accurately measured, provide information on normal biological as well as pathological processes [9, 10], and can change clinical management by guiding shared decision making with patients about risk-reducing strategies [2].

In this chapter, we will discuss the role that biomarkers can play in refining CVD risk estimation for a more individualized approach to prevention. Given the enormity of biomarkers that have been studied over time, this chapter could not be inclusive of all markers; however, it will touch on the major biomarkers that have been investigated in CVD management. This chapter will be divided into 2 major sections—(1) lipid-based biomarkers and (2) non-lipid cardiac biomarkers. The goal is to provide clinicians a framework for best incorporating such biomarkers into clinical care for an individualized approach to CVD prevention and to identify gaps in knowledge that warrant further study.

Lipid Biomarkers and Cardiovascular Risk

An elevated serum cholesterol level was the first biomarker of risk for coronary heart disease (CHD), identified back in the 1961 report from the Framingham Heart Study (FHS) investigators [11]. Since that time, an extensive body of evidence from genetic, epidemiologic, and interventional studies has established elevated low density lipoprotein-cholesterol (LDL-C) as a causal factor for the development of ASCVD [12–14]. Therefore, the management of blood cholesterol for the prevention of ASCVD has become a central focus across clinical guidelines [1, 3, 15]. However, approximately 40% of those who develop CHD do not have elevation in total cholesterol [16]; conversely many individuals with moderately elevated LDL-C do not experience a myocardial infarction (MI) or stroke. Therefore, much work had gone into improving ASCVD risk-estimation beyond cholesterol measurement by considering other traditional ASCVD risk factors, as well as newer "risk-enhancing" factors, to guide shared decision making about implementation of preventive pharmacotherapies (i.e. statins) [2]. Newer lipid measures, as discussed, can provide additional insights into ASCVD risk beyond total cholesterol and the traditionally estimated LDL-C obtained from the Friedewald equation, as well as reflect residual risk despite treatment with statin therapy.

Low-Density Lipoprotein Cholesterol

The development of ASCVD begins with the retention and accumulation of cholesterol-rich apolipoprotein B (apoB)-containing lipoproteins within the arterial intima. Trapping of an atherogenic apoB particle within the vascular wall is the

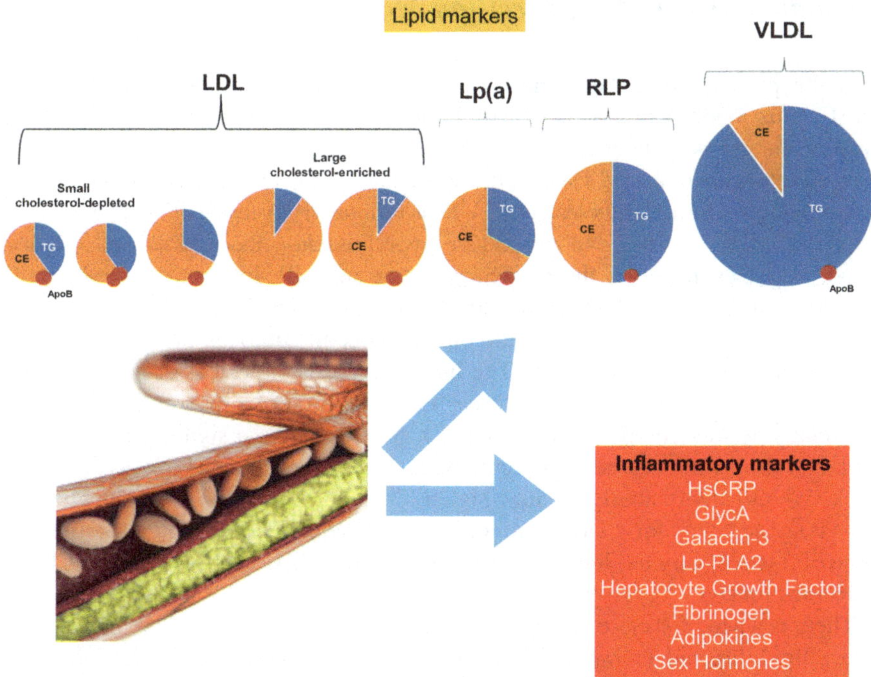

Fig. 1 Lipid and inflammatory markers for development of atherosclerosis

pivotal event that initiates and sustains the atherosclerotic process. Lipoproteins that are highly atherogenic, such as LDL, very low-density lipoprotein (VLDL) and their remnants, intermediate-density lipoprotein (IDL) and lipoprotein (a) (Lp(a)) are small (<70 nm in diameter) and therefore, can easily enter and exit the arterial intima (Fig. 1).

LDL particles represent about 90% of circulating apoB-containing lipoproteins in fasting blood in most individuals. However, concentration of LDL particles in plasma are not routinely measured in clinical practice or used in major randomized clinical trials. Indeed, the total amount of cholesterol carried by these particles, LDL-C, has been broadly used. As the concentrations of LDL-C increase, the probability of retention of LDL in the intima wall increases in a dose-dependent fashion. LDL-C is the most extensively studied modifiable risk factor associated with ASCVD. Prospective cohort studies, Mendelian randomization studies and randomized clinical trials demonstrate a log-linear association between absolute exposure of LDL-C and risk of ASCVD, the so-called "the lower the better" hypothesis [13, 17]. As such, among lipid measures, LDL-C has become the primary focus for assessing and reducing cardiovascular risk, which is supported by guidelines worldwide [1–3, 15].

Estimation of LDL-C in Precision Medicine

Over the past decades, the clinical LDL-C (made up of biological LDL-C plus IDL-C plus lipoprotein (a) [Lp(a)]-C) has been estimated by the Friedewald equation in routine patient care, therefore avoiding additional time and extra costs from direct measurements. The Friedewald equation [Total cholesterol (TC) minus high density lipoprotein-cholesterol (HDL-C) minus triglycerides (TG)/5 in mg/dL units] was derived from 448 normal or hyperlipidemic individuals more than 4 decades ago, even before the existence of current LDL-lowering therapies [18]. However, as Friedewald et al. acknowledged in their original paper, VLDL-C cannot be accurately estimated by the one-size-fits-all approach of dividing TG by the population average value of 5. The inaccuracy was viewed as acceptable at the time because VLDL-C was a relatively small proportion of equation (i.e., VLDL-C was relatively low compared with LDL-C). Subsequently, a significant amount of work has shown the degree of inaccuracy of the Friedewald equation at all LDL-C levels, which is particularly great at higher TG and lower LDL-C levels when the inaccuracy accounts for a larger proportion of the equation [19]. In this setting, the value of 5 is typically too low, and therefore VLDL-C is overestimated, and LDL-C is underestimated.

There is a need for more accurate estimation in the current era where newer more potent lipid-directed therapeutics (such as proprotein convertase subtilisin/kexin type 9 (PCSK9) inhibitors) are reducing LDL-C levels lower than ever seen before. Taking advantage of statistical power of big data, Martin et al. developed and validated a novel method for estimating LDL-C from the standard lipid profile [20]. This method uses 174 different adjustable factors in samples with TG <400 for the TG/VLDL-C ratio based on non-HDL-C and TG levels, and in doing so is an example of a precision medicine rather than one-size-fits-all approach to LDL-C estimation. This approach provides a more accurate estimation of LDL-C, particularly in the setting of low LDL-C and high TG, compared to the Friedewald equation. Elevated TG levels are more relevant nowadays in the current epidemic era of diabetes and obesity. The Martin/Hopkins method has been externally validated in different populations and represents a significant contribution to precision medicine [21–25].

There is More Than LDL-C: LDL Particles and Apolipoprotein B

Each LDL particle contains one single apoB molecule. As stated above, LDL represents ∼90% of apoB-containing lipoproteins. Not surprisingly, lipid-directed therapeutics that lower apoB levels also reduce ASCVD risk, with parallels reductions in LDL-C [26]. However, LDL-C is simply the amount of cholesterol carried by LDL particles (LDL-P). Under most conditions, LDL-C concentration and LDL particle number are highly correlated, and therefore, plasma LDL-C is a good surrogate for LDL particle concentration. However, LDL particles are heterogenous with regards to the mass of cholesterol they carry. As such, LDL particles can be either normal, cholesterol-enriched or cholesterol-depleted. LDL particles contain a normal mass of cholesterol, and only in this situation both LDL-C and LDL-P are *concordant*, and therefore, equivalent markers of cardio-vascular risk. Contrarily, when LDL particles are either cholesterol-enriched or cholesterol-depleted, LDL-C will over- or underrepresent, respectively, the number of LDL particles.

The lipid phenotype of individuals with metabolic conditions such as metabolic syndrome, diabetes or hypertriglyceridemia, is characterized by a predominance of small, dense cholesterol-depleted LDL. In these settings, plasma LDL-C and LDL-P are *discordant* and therefore, plasma LDL-C may not accurately reflect LDL particle concentration or its effect on cardiovascular risk. In these circumstances, direct measurement of LDL-P can more accurately reflect the LDL-related atherogenic burden. However, there are no cost-effective and well standardized measures of LDL-P, and randomized controlled trials have not focused on LDL-P; therefore it remains primarily a research tool.

Most biomarkers are usually assessed at a population level. Lipid parameters, one of the most widely studied biomarkers, can also provide risk information for the general population. Several parameters are now available in lipidology; as more lipid variables are taken into account, the most significant and relevant information obtained can be seen in those with discordance between one and another parameter, and whether this discordance relate to a greater atherosclerosis or greater risk of having events. The real information with regards to risk signals between two lipid parameters that appear to be related (i.e. LDL-C and LDL-P), therefore, should be assessed when they disagree—or are *discordant*—not when they agree. By focusing on these groups, the analysis of discordance can help to more clearly weigh the incremental risk prediction capacity of a given lipid measure over another [27].

Lipid parameters such as LDL-C, non-HDL-C, apoB, and LDL-P are highly correlated one to the other. Most studies aim to compare the predictive power of these variables using conventional statistical methods (i.e. multiple regressions, Cox-proportional hazards) that indeed treat these variables as if they are unrelated, or as if they are expected to provide completely different information like, for instance, age and sex. In order to more accurately discriminate the *additional* information provided by each variable and therefore the real predictive power of each, discordance analyses should be used. Several epidemiologic studies have shown the degree of discordance between LDL-P and LDL-C, and its magnitude on cardiovascular risk prediction. Individuals from the FHS with high LDL-C and high LDL-P, expectedly, had significantly more cardiovascular events than those low LDL-C and low LDL-P. However, the number of events in those with low LDL-C/ high LDL-P did not differ significantly from those with high LDL-C/high LDL-P, which suggests that risk correlates with LDL-P and not with LDL-C [28]. Similarly, a Multi-Ethnic Study of Atherosclerosis (MESA) study showed that whereas both

LDL-C and LDL-P predicted incident cardiovascular events, the risk in the discordant groups was more closely correlated with LDL-P than with LDL-C [29].

A study by Mora et al. of 28,345 women from the Women Health Study (WHS) followed for a mean of 17 years showed a relatively high proportion of discordance (defined by medians) between LDL-C and non-HDL-C (11.6%), LDL-P (24.3%) and apoB (18.9%) [30]. As expected, those with increased number of cholesterol-depleted LDL (or low LDL-C but *discordantly* high LDL-P or apoB) had elevated levels of TG and C-reactive protein, in addition to higher body mass index (BMI). In this *discordant* but highly prevalent group, risk of incident events was greater than in the concordant group with low LDL-C and or low levels of LDL-P or apoB. Additionally, those with cholesterol-enriched apoB particles below the median (high LDL-C but discordantly low LDL-P or apoB) did not have increased risk, which is consistent with previous study from FHS and MESA which also showed that risk is related to particle number rather than to the cholesterol content of apoB particles.

It is important to acknowledge that the definition of discordance is arbitrary as there is no established cut-point at which particles become cholesterol-depleted or cholesterol-enriched. However, multiple studies using different approaches have shown overall same outcomes which provides strong support for the validity of the approach. For instance, a discordance analysis from the Quebec cardiovascular society used quintiles of LDL-C and apoB to define discordance, whereas individuals from the FHS and the WHS were divided into medians [28, 30, 31]. On the other hand, a MESA study defined discordance as ≥ 12 percentile difference between LDL-C and LDL-P [29]. Of note, all these studies have used Friedewald LDL-C instead of more accurate estimation methods. Finally, although these attempts aim to assess existence and relevance of discordance between these lipid markers, all of these cutpoints were arbitrarily estimated from the study populations, and do not have a direct clinical application.

Non-High-Density Lipoprotein Cholesterol (non-HDL-C): The "Poor Man" apoB?

The amount of cholesterol in all non-HDL particles, the so-called non-HDL-C, is simply calculated as TC minus HDL-C. Therefore, no additional measurements need to be done beyond the standard lipid panel. Keeping in mind that TC is the sum of LDL-C + IDL-C + Lp(a)-C + VLDL-C + HDL-C, it could be deduced that non-HDL-C is a better marker of cardiovascular risk than LDL-C because it includes the cholesterol in all atherogenic lipoproteins, in particular LDL-C and VLDL. This becomes particularly important in the presence of hypertriglyceridemia, in which cholesteryl ester can shift from LDL to VLDL in exchange for TG, leading to LDL-C reduction but an increase in VLDL-C. Since these changes are reciprocal and one compensates for the other, non-HDL-C remains unchanged and accounts for the reduction in LDL-C when LDL particles are cholesterol-depleted. However, this hypothesis is not supported by the fact that cholesterol in VLDL particles is not more atherogenic than cholesterol in LDL particles, and VLDL are much larger and less numerous than LDL particles, being less likely to enter the arterial wall [32]. One study from the Framingham Offspring Study showed that adding VLDL particle number does not increase the predictive power of LDL-P, as it should have if the superiority of non-HDL-C over LDL-C was based on including VLDL in the estimate [28]. Additionally, there is not conclusive evidence to date that lowering VLDL-C by means of, for instance, fibrates, lead to benefit.

ApoB particles are present in all atherogenic lipoproteins, where HDL is not included. Therefore, the amount of cholesterol in all non-HDL particles (non-HDL-C) can be a surrogate marker—or indirect measure—of the number of apoB particles. Indeed, these two variables are intimately related physiologically and highly correlated as any change in levels of apoB will lead to changes in cholesterol in non-HDL particles. As proof of this, most studies have shown that the correlation between non-HDL-C and LDL-P or apoB are substantially greater than between LDL-C and LDL-P or apoB, except for one [33].

As expected, both apoB and non-HDL-C appear to be somewhat stronger markers of cardiovascular risk than Friedewald LDL-C. ApoB has been superior to non-HDL-C only in some epidemiological studies, although they have often been equivalent. Whereas non-HDL-C and apoB are highly correlated, they are only moderately concordant because apoB particles differ substantially in the amount of cholesterol they contain [31, 34]. Additionally, statins are known to reduce non-HDL-C more than apoB, for which apoB can better predict risk among statin-treated patients [35]. ApoB and non-HDL-C have been directly compared in the INTERHEART study, which compared 15,512 cases with a first acute MI and 14,820 age and sex-matched controls without known ASCVD from 262 centers in 52 countries [36]. In this study, discordance was defined based on difference in percentile levels (using differences as 1,2,3,4,5 or 10 percentile), and there was an elevated risk in those with high apoB but low non-HDL-C, but decreased in those with low apoB but high non-HDL-C. Another study showed that in a considerable number of individuals, the concentration of apoB and non-HDL-C differed significantly, likely because of variance in their individual metabolism of apoB lipoproteins. Consequently, the individual hazard predicted is also expected to differ [37].

Clinically, two opposite scenarios can be seen:

(A) ApoB > non-HDL-C, which suggests a predominance of cholesterol-depleted LDL particles, and therefore assessment of risk should be driven by apoB [38].
(B) ApoB < non-HDL-C, in which case we should suspect excessive chylomicron and VLDL remnants (type III hyperlipidemia).

Maximizing the Use of the Standard Lipid Panel: The Total Cholesterol to HDL-C Ratio

Total cholesterol and HDL-C are used in ASCVD risk estimating tools (such as the PCE); they are also used for the estimation of LDL-C and calculation of non-HDL-C. Furthermore, the ratio of TC/HDL-C, itself, has been strongly associated with cardiovascular events [39–42]. In a meta-analysis of ~900,000 patients, TC/HDL-C was suggested to have a 40% higher ability to predict vascular deaths than non-HDL-C [43].

Following the advantages of using a discordance approach, the TC/HDL-C ratio could provide additional clinical information to LDL-C or non-HDL-C when discordant with them within individuals. A cross-sectional study of 1.3 million patients, in which discordance was defined as ≥ 25 percentile units difference, ~1 in 3 had discordance between TC/HDL-C and LDL-C, and ~1 in 4 between TC/ HDL-C and non-HDL-C. Patients with low LDL-C or non-HDL-C but with discordantly high TC/HDL-C ratio were more likely to be male, have diabetes, and have a more atherogenic lipid phenotype with lower HDL-C and higher TG [44]. Another study of patients with known coronary artery disease (CAD) showed that the TC/HDL-C ratio reclassified atheroma progression and major adverse cardiovascular event rates in CAD patients when discordant with LDL-C, non-HDL-C and apoB [45]. For instance, among patients with apoB <59 mg/dL, those with discordantly elevated percentile equivalent TC/HDL-C ratio (≥ 2.5) had greater atheroma progression and higher cardiovascular events that those with concordantly low TC/HDL-C ratio (<2.5).

The existence of significant individual-level discordance between the TC/ HDL-C ratio and LDL-C and non-HDL-C was also shown in a large biracial cohort of individuals free from ASCVD at baseline followed for over 20 years. Among those with LDL-C and non-HDL-C < median, 1 in 4 and 1 in 5 had discordantly higher TC/HDL-C $\geq$ median, respectively. They were characterized by higher levels of TGs, higher BMI and more hypertension, diabetes and smoking. Similarly, those with discordance had a significant increase in the risk of incident ASCVD, independent of clinical risk factors and use of lipid-lowering medications [46]. It has been suggested that the TC/HDL-C ratio may reflect the discordance between particle cholesterol content and concentration that frequently is seen in patients with insulin resistance and low HDL-C. As such, the TC/HDL-C may be a marker of atherogenic particle burden with the big advantage that it can be obtained from the standard lipid profile. Previous studies have shown a close association between TC/ HDL-C and LDL-P. A recent analysis showed that TC/HDL-C < 3 was the standard lipid profile measure that was most correlated with LDL-P of <1000 nmol/L [47]. In another study, the significant difference in LDL size between patients with CAD and controls became non-significant after adjusting for TC/HDL-C [48].

In summary, evidence suggests that the TC/HDL-C ratio, available from the standard lipid profile at no extra cost, provides additional information that can enhance personalized ASCVD risk management. Whereas lowering LDL-C is known to reduce risk, lowering the TC/HDL-C ratio could also provide further benefits as the former are cholesterol-based measures which, as discussed above, can underestimate the burden of circulating atherogenic particles. However, whether targeting the TC/HDL-C after optimizing LDL-C can improve patient outcomes is a hypothesis still in need of testing in randomized controlled trials.

Residual Risk and Lipoprotein-Related Risk Beyond LDL: Triglyceride-Rich Lipoproteins

Triglycerides have had growing interest as a target of ASCVD prevention, because of their consistent causal association with ASCVD and their increased levels associated with obesity [49, 50]. Lifestyle measures—reduced intake of simple refined carbohydrates and alcohol, increased physical activity, and weight loss—remain the first-line treatment for elevated TG, with statin therapy added for ASCVD prevention for those at elevated ASCVD risk (secondary prevention and high risk primary prevention) [15]. Furthermore, the 2019 ACC/AHA Guideline on the Primary Prevention of CVD states that persistently elevated TG >175 mg/dL (non-fasting, on ≥ 3 occasions) is considered a "risk-enhancing" factor that would also favor statin treatment among those at estimated borderline/intermediate ASCVD risk [2].

More recently, TG have been of particular interest as a treatment target because of their relationship with residual risk for ASCVD among statin-treated individuals. Schwartz et al. examined the association between fasting TG levels with recurrent ASCVD in statin-treated participants from the Myocardial Ischemia Reduction with Aggressive Cholesterol Lowering (MIRACL) and dal-OUTCOMES trials [51, 52]. They found a 50–60% increase in hazard for recurrent events among those in the highest TG categories compared with those in the lowest, after adjustment for several risk factors and independent of LDL-C [53]. A post-hoc analysis from the Pravastatin or Atorvastatin Evaluation and Infection Therapy–Thrombolysis in Myocardial Infarction 22 (PROVE IT-TIMI 22) trial showed a reduction in recurrent events with lower on-treatment TG levels in statin-treated participants, independent of LDL-C [54].

With the exception of icosapent ethyl [55] (discussed below), other trials that have evaluated TG-lowering pharmacotherapies (i.e. fibrates, niacin) to reduce residual risk beyond statin therapy have been disappointing. However, post-hoc analyses from the Action to Control Cardiovascular Risk in Diabetes (ACCORD) and the Atherothrombosis Intervention in Metabolic Syndrome with Low HDL/High Triglycerides: Impact on Global Health Outcomes (AIM-HIGH) trial showed that fibrates and niacin, respectively, would provide benefit only in the subgroup with elevated TG and low HDL-C, for which it was thought that elevated TG would help to better identify patients in whom residual risk could be further reduced [56, 57]. More recently, the Reduction of Cardiovascular Events with Icosapent Ethyl–Intervention Trial (REDUCE-IT) showed a significant reduction in cardiovascular events among statin-treated individuals with elevated TG (>135 mg/dL) who received 4 g of icosapent ethyl daily (a highly purified form of eicosapentaenoic acid (EPA)), although this benefit appeared to be independent of baseline or achieved TG levels, suggesting non-lipid mechanisms for its benefit [55]. Furthermore, this may be specific to EPA as other omega-3 preparations, such as docosahexaenoic acid (DHA)/ EPA combination, have not shown CVD benefit [58]. As novel TG-lowering therapies are being developed, such as antisense inhibition of APOC3 synthesis, it is expected that elevated TG levels will become progressively more clinically relevant to identify individuals that would benefit from these therapies [59].

Indeed, a number of Mendelian randomization and prospective studies have supported a causal role for TG-rich remnants in atherosclerosis [60–63]. In a cohort of 5,754 statin-treated patients with CAD undergoing serial intravascular ultrasonography, remnant cholesterol was associated with residual risk independent of conventional lipid parameters, C-reactive protein (CRP) or clinical risk factors [64]. Although it is extensively known how LDL particles and LDL cholesterol contribute to atherosclerosis, the atherogenic properties of remnants are not fully understood [65]. Finally, despite given ongoing interest for remnant cholesterol and residual risk, there is a need to standardize its definitions and measurements [66].

Lipoprotein (a)—ready for Prime-Time Use?

Lipoprotein (a) , or Lp(a), is a cholesterol-rich, LDL-like particle with an apoB-100 covalently bound by a disulfide bond to apolipoprotein (a), mostly genetically determined by the LPA gene, that has well described atherogenic properties, as well as theoretical but unproven prothrombotic properties [67]. Mounting evidence, from epidemiologic, Mendelian randomization and genome-wide association studies, supports the causal association of elevated Lp(a) and development of ASCVD [68–75].

Some studies have suggested a potential role of Lp(a) for risk assessment. In the Bruneck study, 15-year primary prevention cohort, Lp(a) improved both risk discrimination and reclassification when added to Framingham and Reynolds Risk Scores (up to 39.6% in the intermediate risk group) [76]. In the European Prospective Investigation of Cancer (EPI)—Norfolk cohort, adding Lp(a) (<dichotomized as <30 and ≥ 30 mg/dL) to both the PCE and SCORE risk estimators resulted in net reclassification index (NRI) of 15.9 and 16.8%, respectively, among intermediate risk individuals [77]. In the Copenhagen City Heart Study, addition of elevated Lp(a) (≥ 50 mg/dL) to conventional CVD risk factors yielded a NRI of 16% for MI and 3% for CAD [78]. The Brisighella Heart Study found that Lp(a) was a significant predictor of CVD over 25 years in those with intermediate or high risk [79]. Among patients with established CAD, Lp(a) was a significant independent predictor of recurrent CVD, either in non-obstructive CAD, as well as patients undergoing percutaneous coronary interventions and those treated with statin therapy [80, 81].

Although statins do not reduce Lp(a) levels, and may even increase Lp(a) modestly, among high risk patients with elevated Lp(a), statin therapy still remains first line for overall ASCVD risk reduction [1]. Other lipid-lowering therapies have been shown to mild to moderately reduce Lp(a) levels. Niacin has been shown to reduce Lp(a) but not CVD events [75, 82]. However, it is important to note that none of the niacin trials selected patients based on elevated Lp(a). In the Further Cardiovascular Outcomes Research with PCSK9 Inhibition in Subjects with Elevated Risk (FOURIER) trial, evolocumab reduced Lp(a) by a median of 27% at 48 weeks. Interestingly, those with Lp(a) above the median at baseline had a 23% relative risk reduction in CAD. Furthermore, there was a significant relationship between achieved Lp(a) at 12 weeks and adjusted risk of events [72].

Given the current lack of Lp(a)-targeted therapies, the case for Lp(a) screening has been questioned by experts and in this scenario, recent guidelines differ slightly in their recommendations. The 2018 AHA/ACC Cholesterol Management Guideline recognizes Lp(a) as a "risk enhancer" in adults between the ages of 40 to 75 years, in whom those with Lp(a) $\geq$ 50 mg/dL would be favored to start statin therapy [1]. However, limited guidance is given as to when Lp(a) should be measured; family history of premature CAD or personal history of ASCVD not explained by major risk factors are relative indications for measurement. In contrast, the European Society of Cardiology (ESC)/European Atherosclerosis Society (EAS) guidelines recommend that all adults have Lp(a) measured at least once in their lifetime to identify those with very high Lp(a) > 180 mg/dL who have a lifetime risk similar to those with heterozygous familial hypercholesterolemia, and should be measured selectively among those with a family history of premature CAD or at borderline/intermediate risk to revise their risk estimation [3].

Despite compelling evidence for the causal role of Lp(a) in ASCVD risk, evidence is lacking that specifically lowering Lp(a) leads to a meaningful reduction in cardiovascular events, which continues to limit its clinical use. One Mendelian analysis demonstrated that while the clinical benefit of Lp(a) lowering is proportional to the reduction in Lp(a) concentration, large absolute reductions ($\sim$ 100 mg/dL) are necessary to produce a clinically meaningful impact on cardiovascular outcomes [83]. A recent phase 2 randomized clinical trial showed that the hepatocyte-directed antisense oligonucleotide APO(a)-L$_{RX}$ reduced Lp(a) levels in a dose-dependent manner to up to 80% [73]. The phase 3 study is ongoing (NCT04023552) and, if such Lp(a) reduction translates into reduction of ASCVD clinical outcomes, it is expected that screening for Lp(a) its use in ASCVD risk estimation will continue to gain relevance and be ready for prime-time clinical use.

From the laboratory measurement standpoint, there are two main issues that impact the implementation of Lp(a) in clinical practice. First, most assays report Lp(a) values as mass concentrations (mg/dL) instead of particle concentrations (nmol/L). Second, there are no standardized Lp(a) assays [84].

Non-Lipid Cardiac Biomarkers in Risk Stratification of Asymptomatic Patients

In this second section, we will discuss biomarkers of wall stress (natriuretic peptides), of myocardial injury (troponins) (section **A**), and inflammation (hsCRP, GlycA) (section **B**), as well as other novel/emerging biomarkers under investigation (section **C**) (Fig. 1).

A. Troponin and Natriuretic Peptides

Cardiac Biomarkers of Wall Stress and Myocardial Injury

Two of the most studied groups of cardiac biomarkers are the myofibrillar protein cardiac troponin (cTn) and the natriuretic peptide derivatives such as B-type natriuretic peptide (BNP) and its amino-terminal cleavage equivalent (NT-proBNP) (Fig. 2). While these biomarkers have traditionally been used to identify symptomatic cardiac pathology such as acute coronary syndrome and decompensated heart failure (HF), their presence in asymptomatic individuals also has important implications for risk stratification.

Cardiac troponins are regulatory proteins that control the interactions between actin and myosin necessary for contraction of cardiomyocytes [85]. In the setting of oxygen supply/demand imbalance at cardiomyocytes, myocardial ischemia and necrosis occurs, resulting in elevation of cardiac troponins in the blood. Importantly, these elevations can occur with both clinical and sub-clinical myocardial injury. With the advent of high-sensitivity troponin (hs-cTn) assays,

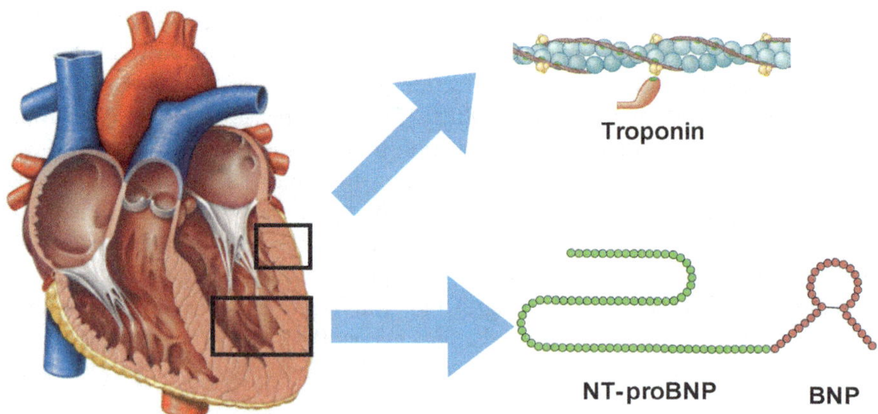

Fig. 2 Cardiac biomarkers of wall stress and myocardial injury

cardiac troponins can be measured above the limit of detection in $\geq 50\%$ of overtly normal individuals [86]. High-sensitivity assays for troponin T and I (hs-cTnT and hs-cTnI) have the potential to identify patients with asymptomatic myocardial injury who may be at increased risk of disease progression.

BNP and NT-proBNP are released into the circulation from ventricular myocardium in the setting of increased end-diastolic wall stress from increased volume or pressure [87]. These natriuretic peptides have diuretic, natriuretic, and hypotensive effects, and contribute to the body's physiologic response to HF [88]. Given their presence in these pathologic states, assays for both BNP and NT-proBNP are widely used. As a surrogate of ventricular wall stress, these natriuretic peptides are clinically useful biomarkers. When used alongside of clinical symptoms and exam findings, natriuretic peptides can help establish diagnosis of acute onset of HF to distinguish it from other causes of dyspnea such as chronic obstructive pulmonary disease exacerbations. Natriuretic peptides can also be used among asymptomatic individuals to identify those with subclinical disease at risk for developing HF who may benefit from more intensive risk-factor modification and further diagnostic evaluation.

Factors Affecting Biomarker Interpretation

It is important to acknowledge certain patient characteristics that can affect interpretation of these biomarkers. Particularly, patients with kidney failure can have persistently elevated troponin, BNP, and NT-proBNP levels regardless of cardiac pathology [89, 90]. This can complicate a biomarker's prognostic value, as cut-off values in end-stage kidney disease are less well defined. A patient's age and sex also affect these biomarkers [91]. Conventionally, the upper limit of normal for hs-cTnT assays is defined as the 99th percentile, which in a normal reference population was found to be 14 ng/L; however, subsequent population based studies have shown that the 99th percentile value may be higher in older patients and in men, leading to over-diagnosis of cardiac pathology in these groups [92]. Sex-specific thresholds of hs-cTn have been proposed for the evaluation of myocardial injury [93]. In community cohorts, women have higher BNP and NT-proBNP than men [91]. High BNP values are also seen among older individuals [94]. BNP cutoffs for subclinical and acute HF are 10 pmol/L and 29 pmol/L respectively; however, age- and sex-specific cut-offs in BNP reference ranges could lead to more a patient specific risk assessment.

Lack of standardization across biomarker assays also complicates interpretation. While a single troponin T assay exists, there are several troponin I assays that vary in their limit of detection, absolute troponin values, and variance within the assay [95]. The International Federation of Clinical Chemistry and Laboratory Medicine Working Group on Standardization of cTnI (IFCC WG-TNI) is in the process of developing a reference immunoassay measurement procedure for troponin I that commercial assays could be calibrated against [96]. There are similar concerns with natriuretic peptide assays, as marked differences in analytic performance and measured values exists between the several commercially available assays for BNP and NT-proBNP [97].

Cardiac Troponin and Cardiovascular Risk

Population based studies have shown that elevations in cardiac troponins are associated with adverse clinical outcomes. In an investigation of the Dallas Heart Study (DHS) cohort, high levels of hs-cTn were associated with increased prevalence of left ventricular hypertrophy, and subsequent all-cause mortality [98]. This predictive value may be stronger in patients with higher baseline cardiovascular risk. The Troponina T UltraSensible en pacientes Asintomáticos de alto Riesgo Cardiovascular (TUSARC) study investigated the prognostic value of elevated hs-cTnT in an asymptomatic Spanish population characterized as high-risk by ESC Guidelines [99]. This study found that an elevation in hs-cTnT greater than the 99th percentile was significantly associated with the incidence of a combined outcome of death by cardiovascular cause, HF requiring hospitalization or intravenous diuretics, non-fatal stroke, non-fatal acute coronary syndrome, or the need for coronary revascularization. Minimal elevation in troponin less than the upper limit of normal may also have prognostic value. In the West of Scotland Coronary Prevention Study (WOSCOPS), an elevated baseline hs-cTnI (less than the 99th percentile) was shown to be an independent predictor of MI or death from CHD in male patients with elevated LDL-C levels. Furthermore statin therapy reduced hs-cTnI and those with greater reduction in hs-cTnI had lower CAD risk [100]. In an Atherosclerosis Risk in Communities (ARIC) study, among individuals free of CVD at baseline, an elevated hs-cTnI $\geq$ 3.8 ng/L was associated with subsequent risk of incident CAD, stroke, HF, and total CVD [101]. Furthermore, the addition of hs-cTnT to the PCE improved risk CVD prediction compared to the PCE alone [101]. Given this prognostic value, novel risk calculators have incorporated hs-cTn measurements in determining future cardiovascular risk; this approach is especially helpful in older patients, who may be re-classified into a lower risk category and spared more aggressive medical therapies [102].

Of note the 2019 ACC/AHA Primary Prevention Guideline does not specifically acknowledge hs-cTn as a risk enhancing factor for treatment decisions [2]. This may change in future as further evidence accumulates to support its role a decision aide tool for guiding pharmacotherapy. Given the prognostic value of these biomarkers, several studies have already investigated the utility of a biomarker-based approach in the risk-stratification and management of patients. The following discussion highlights the utility of hs-cTn and natriuretic peptide measurement in the management of several common cardiac pathologies.

Cardiac Biomarkers in Hypertension

Hypertension is one of the most common cardiac comorbidities, and exhibits a wide spectrum of severity and symptomatology. Given hypertension's associated morbidity and mortality, the identification of patients at increased risk of incident hypertension through biomarkers can be of clinical benefit. A study in the ARIC cohort showed that among patients free from CVD, a baseline elevation in hs-cTn was associated with development of hypertension and left ventricular hypertrophy over 20 years of follow-up [103]. This study suggests that identification of low risk, normotensive patients with elevated hs-cTn could afford clinicians the opportunity to consider ambulatory blood pressure monitoring, or more intensive prevention strategies.

A biomarker-based approach could also identify patients with increased risk of cardiovascular events due to hypertension in whom treatment decisions are unclear. For example, in the 2017 ACC/AHA Blood Pressure Guideline states than patients with an elevated blood pressure (120 to 129/ <80 mm Hg) or low-risk stage 1 hypertension (130 to 139/80 to 89 mm Hg) are not recommended for antihypertensive medication; therefore, management of these patients can prove challenging, as they carry increased risk without a clear indication for medical therapy. However, one study using pooled data from the ARIC, DHS, and MESA cohorts showed that 32% of individuals in this group had elevated hs-cTn or NT-proBNP. In these individuals not recommended for medical therapy, the presence of biomarker elevation was associated with an 11% incidence rate of ASCVD or HF, compared to 4.6% in those without elevated biomarkers [104]. Conversely, among individuals who were recommended for anti-hypertensive therapy, more than half had a non-elevated hs-cTn and NT-proBNP; lack of biomarker elevation was associated with a less than 10% risk of cardiovascular event. Notably, the authors still favor initiating anti-hypertensive therapy in these patients given the cost-effectiveness and proven utility of medical therapy, but suggest that biomarker measurement may be useful in informing the shared decision making process.

Cardiac Biomarkers in Aortic Stenosis

Another high-mortality cardiac pathology that may benefit from a biomarker-based approach is aortic stenosis. Aortic stenosis (AS) is the most common form of valvular heart disease in the developed world, and symptomatic AS is associated with significant morbidity and mortality. While asymptomatic AS is traditionally not intervened upon until symptoms develop, recent studies have challenged this thinking [105]. The ESC and European Association of Cardio-thoracic surgery recommends that aortic valve replacement may be considered in asymptomatic patients with severe AS who have a normal ejection fraction, low surgical risk, and marked elevation in natriuretic peptide levels confirmed by repeated measurements and without other explanation [106]. Studies have also investigated the utility of hs-cTn as a useful tool in AS management. As cardiomyocyte damage is a late event in the natural progression of AS, hs-cTn may serve as a more specific marker of clinically significant AS when compared to BNP [107]. One study showed elevated hs-cTnI levels in patients with AS were associated with need for aortic valve replacement independent of age, sex, systolic ejection fraction, or AS severity [108]. Another study measured hs-cTn levels in 58 patients with asymptomatic severe AS, and found a hs-cTnT level greater than 10 ng/L was associated with an approximately tenfold increase in the composite outcome of cardiovascular death, new-onset symptoms, cardiac hospitalization, guideline-driven indication for valve replacement and cardiovascular death at 12 months [109]. Given this association, novel risk calculators predicting adverse outcomes in AS have begun to incorporate hs-cTn levels [110].

Cardiac Biomarkers in Heart Failure

The clinical syndrome of HF is the end stage of several cardiovascular conditions. Given the heterogeneity of HF causes, it can be difficult to predict incident HF in the general population. In the FHS, baseline elevation in BNP and urinary albumin to creatinine ratio was associated with increased risk for the development of new-onset HF [111]. Elevated troponin levels are also seen across the clinical spectrum of HF, with up to 50–80% of patients with asymptomatic HF having hs-cTn levels above the limit of detection [112]. In an ARIC study of individuals without CVD or HF at baseline, hs-cTnT levels ≥ 3.8 ng/L was associated with a fourfold risk of incident HF hospitalization over 15 years [HR 4.20 (95% CI 3.25–5.37)] [101].

A few prospective studies have explored the utility of a biomarker-based approach to HF management. The St Vincent's Screening to Prevent Heart Failure trial randomized 1374 patients with elevated cardiovascular risk to either usual primary care or screening with BNP testing. Patients in the screening arm found to have BNP levels greater than 50 pg/mL underwent echocardiography and collaborative care with cardiologist input, which often lead to more intensive risk factor control and medical therapy. This BNP based screening approach was shown to reduce the combined rates of LV systolic dysfunction, diastolic dysfunction, and HF [113]. Similarly, the Screening Evaluation of the Evolution of New Heart Failure (SCREEN-HF) study examined NT-proBNP levels in patients with high cardiovascular risk but without prevalent HF; patients with NT-proBNP at the highest quintile (>30 pmol/L) were found to have higher rates of left ventricular systolic impairment and higher potential risk of incident HF [114]. Given this data, a recent AHA statement indicated that in community-based populations, measurement of natriuretic peptides or troponins alone adds prognostic information to standard risk factors for predicting new-onset HF [115].

As assays for troponins and natriuretic peptides continue to evolve, so too will their role in the risk stratification of asymptomatic patients. Professional societies have begun to recognize their utility in predicting incident CVD, and it is possible that future recommendations will further expand the role of these commonly available assays.

B. Inflammatory Markers

Inflammation plays a key role in the development of atherosclerosis and thrombosis [116, 117]. High-sensitivity C-reactive protein (hsCRP) and other inflammatory biomarkers can predict risk for ASCVD events independently of traditional risk factors [118]. Lifestyle measures such as weight loss, physical activity, and smoking cessation are central for reducing the inflammatory risk associated with cardio-metabolic diseases. Regarding pharmacotherapy, the efficacy of statin therapy in reducing ASCVD risk may in part be due to their anti-inflammatory properties, though recent studies suggest the benefit of this pleotropic effect is minimal compared to the impact of lowering LDL-C [119, 120]. Among individuals with elevated hsCRP levels ≥ 2 mg/L, but with low LDL-C <130 mg/dL, rosuvastatin conferred a 44% reduction in major adverse cardiac events in the Justification for the Use of Statins in Prevention: an Intervention Trial Evaluating Rosuvastatin (JUPITER) trial [121]. As proof of concept for causality of inflammation in ASCVD pathogenesis, the Canakinumab Anti-inflammatory Thrombosis Outcome Study (CANTOS) showed that an anti-inflammatory therapy targeting interleukin-1β reduced the risk of recurrent CVD events independently of lipid-lowering [122]. Thus, inflammatory markers have appeal as both prognostic markers of risk and also therapeutic targets.

HsCRP

High-sensitivity C-reactive protein has emerged as the most commonly utilized marker of systemic inflammation in clinical practice. hsCRP has been shown to be associated with incident CVD events, independent of traditional risk factors [118, 123, 124]. In the ARIC study, an elevated hsCRP greater than the median (≥ 2.4 mg/L) was associated with an increased ~ 30–50% ASCVD risk, even among individuals who had low cholesterol defined by having multiple measures of atherogenic lipid particles below the median [124]. Some risk estimator tools, notably the Reynolds Risk Score, have incorporated hsCRP in their models, with improvement in re-classification of risk [125, 126].

While hsCRP appears may be a useful prognostic marker of risk, whether to use hsCRP levels as a treatment goal remains a matter of controversy [127–129]. Post-hoc analyses of the JUPITER [130], Pravastatin or Atorvastatin Evaluation and Infection Therapy trial (PROVE-IT) TIMI-22 [131], and Improved Reduction of Outcomes: Vytorin Efficacy International Trial (IMPROVE-IT) [132] trials showed that individuals who achieved both the dual goals of low LDL-C <70 mg/ dL and low hsCRP <2 mg/L experienced lower ASCVD event rates compared to those who did not achieve these dual goals. Similarly in the CANTOS trial, the benefit of canakinumab on lowering ASCVD events was seen only among those who achieved on-treatment of hsCRP < 2 mg/L at 3 months but not those who remained with levels ≥ 2 mg/L on-treatment [133]. However, individuals who achieved lower hsCRP on therapy also started with lower hsCRP levels at baseline and had more favorable CVD risk profiles; thus, residual confounding may still explain the associations seen [128, 129]. Additionally, while inflammation is involved in the pathogenesis of atherosclerosis, hsCRP is a non-specific measurement of inflammation, and is not itself involved in the causal pathway of ASCVD. At this time, the 2018 AHA/ACC Cholesterol Guideline (1) and the 2019 ACC/AHA Primary Prevention Guideline (2) endorse using hsCRP (if measured) as a "risk-enhancing factor" that would favor the initiation or intensification of statin therapy among those at borderline or intermediate risk; but they do not endorse following hsCRP levels on treatment or targeting specific hsCRP goals.

GlycA

GlycA is a composite biomarker of systemic inflammation measured by nuclear magnetic resonance (NMR) and reflects the serum concentration and glycosylation state of main acute-phase reactants such as α1-acid glycoprotein, haptoglobin, α1-antitrypsin, α1-antichymotrypsin and transferrin [134]. Compared with hsCRP, this biomarker has several advantages, including its composite nature, lower intra-individual variability, and improved analytic precision [134].

Several epidemiology studies have found elevated plasma GlycA to be associated with increased risk for incident CVD events and all-cause mortality, even after adjustment for other inflammatory markers such as hsCRP [123, 135–140]. GlycA was associated with HF with preserved ejection fraction, even after accounting for adiposity [140]. Among individuals without clinical CVD, plasma GlycA levels were associated with poorer cardiovascular health [141] and with several measures of subclinical atherosclerosis [142–144]. Therefore, GlycA appears to hold promise as a prognostic marker of risk, although it was not specifically listed in the 2019 ACC/AHA Primary Prevention Guideline for this purpose [2]. Whether therapeutic lowering of GlycA (by lifestyle or pharmacotherapy) can prevent CVD remains uncertain. This warrants further study before there can be clinical adoption of GlycA measurement for the purposes of risk assessment, management, or follow-up of patients.

C. **Other Novel Biomarkers of CVD Risk**

The field of biomarkers is continually evolving, with several novel biomarkers currently under investigation. While studies have shown a prognostic value for these biomarkers, further research is needed to fully elucidate their utility in risk stratification and cardiovascular disease prevention.

Galectin-3

Galectin-3 has been linked with cell fibrosis, inflammation, and myocardial remodeling. Macrophages released during myocardial stress are a major source of galectin-3, which may modulate the inflammatory response of damaged cardiac tissue [145]. Rat models have shown that high levels of galectin-3 may be linked to the development of HF, and galectin-3 knockout mice exhibited less fibrosis and better echocardiographic parameters of cardiac function in the setting of pressure overload [146]. Population studies have also shown that galectin-3 may have prognostic value in risk stratification; the Prevention of REnal and Vascular ENd-stage Disease (PREVEND) study showed galectin-3 levels are correlated with many traditional cardiovascular risk factors, including blood pressure, serum lipids, BMI, kidney function, and NT-proBNP [147]. High galectin-3 levels in this population were also associated with increased all-cause mortality. Given this association, galectin-3 was approved by U.S. Food and Drug Administration in 2010 as a new biomarker in the risk stratification of HF. However, it should be noted that in the ARIC cohort, elevated galectin-3 was associated with incident HF only in whites, not blacks, suggesting racial differences in the processes by which galectin-3 confers disease [148].

Lp-PLA2

Lipoprotein-associated phospholipase A2 (Lp-PLA2) plays a critical role in metabolizing pro-inflammatory phospholipids and in the generation of pro-atherogenic metabolites [149]. Multiple studies have shown that elevated Lp-PLA2 levels have prognostic value. A study of the ARIC population showed that Lp-PLA2 was an independent predictor of CHD [150] and also might add additional risk prognostication among individuals who are current smokers [151]. The JUPITER study showed patients in the fourth quartile of Lp-PLA2 levels had a two-fold increased risk of cardiovascular events compared to patients in the first quartile [152]. Based on these data, several professional societies note the measurement of Lp-PLA2 has value in risk stratification for asymptomatic patients, particularly those at moderate cardiovascular risk [153]. However, the more recent 2019 ACC/AHA Guideline for Primary Prevention of CVD only highlights hsCRP as a risk-enhancing factor and does not specifically mention Lp-PLA2 [2]. This may be because while the association between high Lp-PLA2 levels and cardiovascular risk has been demonstrated, the clinical utility of this biomarker remains unclear [154]. A randomized trial failed to show the benefit of the Lp-PLA2 inhibitor darapladib in coronary artery disease, casting some doubt on Lp-PLA2's causal role in atherogenesis [155].

Hepatocyte Growth Factor

Hepatocyte growth factor (HGF) is an angiogenic growth factor expressed in endothelial and vascular smooth muscle cells [156], and thought to have many potentially favorable mechanisms, such as being anti-apoptotic, angiogenic, anti-fibrotic, and anti-inflammatory. In mouse models of HF, HGF reduces adverse ventricular remodeling following an ischemic insult [157]. HGF is released in circulation in response to endothelial damage, [158] and so while its physiologic function is thought to be favorable, HGF elevation in the blood is marker of increased risk for CVD [159–161], likely reflecting compensatory states that ultimately proved inadequate.

In the MESA study, elevated levels of HGF were an independent predictor of incident CHD [158], stroke [161], and progression of atherosclerosis [162, 163]. HGF has also been associated with incident HF with preserved ejection fraction [164] and with a more concentric pattern of left ventricular remodeling [165]. Higher HGF levels have been associated with increased mortality risk among patients with advanced HF [166]. Additionally, high levels of HGF have been associated with traditional risk factors of hypertension, obesity, and diabetes [167]. Measurement of HGF is currently not endorsed in any professional guidelines at this time, and additional studies are necessary to determine its clinical utility in risk stratification.

Fibrinogen

Fibrinogen is a clotting factor and acute phase reactant involved in platelet aggregation, endothelial injury, plasma viscosity, and thrombus formation. The Fibrinogen Studies Collaboration showed that high fibrinogen levels are associated with incident CHD, stroke, and other vascular mortality [168]. The 2012 ESC Guidelines on CVD Prevention allowed for the measurement of fibrinogen in the risk assessment of unusual or moderate risk of cardiovascular disease, but not in asymptomatic low-risk patients; notably, this recommendation was not carried forward into the 2016 guidelines [169, 170]. The 2019 ACC/AHA Primary Prevention Guideline also does not list fibrinogen as one of the risk enhancing factors [2].

Adipokines

Adipose tissue has an important endocrine role in the body through the production of bioactive products known as adipokines. Obesity is characterized by an increase in visceral fat, which leads to an imbalance in adipokines and many of the endocrine and endovascular complications seen in the metabolic syndrome [171], which in turn may increase risk for CVD [172]. Multiple studies have reported an association between adipokines with incident diabetes [173] and ASCVD [174–177], and these associations have been independent of BMI. Adipokines have also been implicated in gestational diabetes, [178] and dysregulation of adipokines during pregnancy may be one mechanism linking multi-parity to future CVD risk in women [179].

One of the most studied adipokines is adiponectin; while it is produced by adipose tissue, it is paradoxically low in obese patients and may have a protective effect on inflammation and atherosclerosis by decreasing monocyte adhesion to endothelial cells and promoting angiogenesis [180]. Adiponectin is thought to have favorable vasodilatory, anti-apoptotic, anti-inflammatory, and anti-oxidative properties. However, studies on adiponectin as a biomarker for risk stratification of CVD have shown mixed results. One prior study showed that patients in the highest quintile of adiponectin levels have a significantly decreased risk of MI compared to those in the lowest quintile, even after adjustment for LDL-C, HDL-C, BMI, history of diabetes and hypertension [175]. However, a subsequent study of the British Regional Heart Study did not show a statistically significant association between adiponectin levels and subsequent CHD [181]. This discrepancy may be due to over-adjustment for other associated biomarkers such as cholesterol levels and inflammatory markers, and additional studies will be necessary to further clarify the role of adiponectin in risk stratification.

Leptin was the first adipokine to be characterized in 1994; it is felt to be pro-atherogenic by initiating leukocyte and macrophage recruitment to the endothelial cell wall and increasing oxidative stress [171]. Disruption of leptin signaling could lead to cardiac hypertrophy [182]. In the FHS, increased levels of leptin were shown to be associated with incident HF [183]. However, a study of the MESA population showed that elevated leptin levels were not associated with incident cardiovascular events [177].

Elevated resistin is thought to promote insulin resistance, inflammation, endothelial dysfunction, foam cell formation, and thrombosis [184]. In the MESA study there was an independent association between higher resistin levels and incident CHD, CVD, and HF [174].

In addition to adiponectin, leptin, and resistin there are several additional adipokines that may serve as biomarkers of CVD, including visfatin, apelin, omentin, and chemerin [171]. While studies in animal models have shown a correlation between these peptides and CVD, additional research is needed to better understand their potential role in clinical risk stratification. Despite their associations with cardiometabolic diseases, at this time, adipokine measurement is not widely used in clinical practice for ASCVD risk prediction or treatment monitoring, and was not specifically mentioned in the 2019 ACC/AHA Primary Prevention Guideline as one of the "risk enhancers".

Sex Hormones

Favorable properties of endogenous estrogens in pre-menopausal women have been implicated as one of the mechanisms to explain the average onset of CAD approximately 10-years later in women on average compared to men. Early menopause is an independent risk for incident ASCVD in women [185], and also mentioned as one of the "risk enhancing" factors in the 2019 ACC/AHA Guideline [2]. The post-menopausal ovary continues to make testosterone, and higher androgen levels in post-menopausal women (i.e., a more "male-like" hormone pattern) has been associated with increased risk for CVD events [186]. In post-menopausal women, higher free testosterone levels have been associated with adverse left ventricular remodeling, aortic stiffness, endothelial dysfunction, subclinical atherosclerosis progression, and increased NT-proBNP [91, 187–190]. Whereas, higher DHEA levels may be associated with decreased risk for ASCVD and HF [191]. Conversely, in men, low testosterone levels have been associated with increased CVD and mortality risk [192, 193]. Despite the fact that sex hormone levels may identify a higher risk individual, sex hormone levels are not measured clinically for the purpose of CVD risk stratification. This is likely because at this time hormone replacement therapy in women and testosterone therapy in men are not recommended for the purposes of ASCVD risk reduction. However, hormone therapy might be used for other indications such as for menopausal vasomotor symptoms or low libido, respectively, in otherwise low risk women and men.

Conclusions

In sum, biomarkers measured from serum or plasma include markers in the direct causal pathway of ASCVD risk, as well as markers that capture subclinical signs of wall stress or myocardial damage, detect inflammatory states, or reflect compensatory states in response to vascular injury. Risk estimation tools incorporating traditional risk factors alone, such as the PCE, are imprecise [6, 194]. These calculators estimate the average risk in a group of individuals who have similar risk factor profiles, but a given risk score is far more accurate for populations than it is for any particular individual [4, 5]. Therefore assessment of biomarkers, alongside of traditional CVD risk factors, has the potential to provide a more personalized assessment of risk for a given individual. However, with the array of biomarkers to choose from, the question arises of which marker or panel of markers has the most prognostic utility in guiding shared decision making for implementing preventive pharmacotherapies. Many of these biomarkers do not sufficiently change the area under the curve (C-statistics) over traditional risk factors and as such have not been endorsed for routine CVD risk assessment. Furthermore, it has also been questioned about whether biomarkers have any benefit over direct assessment of atherosclerosis such as the CAC score [195–198].

At this time, current 2019 ACC/AHA Guideline for the Primary Prevention of CVD has highlighted elevated hsCRP, TGs, apoB, and Lp(a) as the most helpful "risk-enhancing" factors, that if measured, would favor initiation or intensification of statin therapy among borderline or intermediate risk individuals. In high risk primary prevention or secondary prevention, these lipid markers capture residual risk despite statin therapy and could potentially be used to guide add-on therapies (PCSK9 inhibitors, icosapent ethyl, or novel lipid therapeutics currently under investigation) for further ASCVD risk reduction. Examples include use of icosapent ethyl for elevated TGs despite controlled LDL-C, and PCSK9 inhibitor may be considered to reduce Lp(a) in secondary prevention populations at very high risk. It is important to acknowledge that further studies will be needed to support approaches that are not included in the current guidelines. Additionally, natriuretic peptides and high-sensitivity troponin assays are also increasingly being incorporated into clinical practice to guide clinical management decisions such as in HF and AS, as mentioned above.

On the other hand, some of the other biomarkers mentioned in this review are not commonly used despite showing initial promise of prognostic markers of CVD risk, as it is not clear how management decisions should be changed after their measurement among asymptomatic individuals. Despite the growing body of evidence at the *population*-level supporting a link between these markers and development of CVD, a better characterization of the accuracy of each of them at an *individual*-level and how they can be used to tailor therapy is needed to facilitate their implementation in clinical practice in the era of precision medicine. Future studies should focus on whether biomarker-directed management strategies can improve clinical outcomes compared traditional risk factors approaches alone.

References

1. Grundy SM, Stone NJ, Bailey AL, Beam C, Birtcher KK, Blumenthal RS, et al. 2018 AHA/ACC/AACVPR/AAPA/ABC/ACPM/ADA/AGS/APhA/ASPC/NLA/PCNA guideline on the management of blood cholesterol: executive summary: a report of the American college of cardiology/American heart association task force on clinical practice guidelines. Circulation. 2019;139(25):e1046–81.
2. Arnett DK, Blumenthal RS, Albert MA, Buroker AB, Goldberger ZD, Hahn EJ, et al. 2019 ACC/AHA guideline on the primary prevention of cardiovascular disease: a report of the American college of cardiology/American heart association task force on clinical practice guidelines. Circulation. 2019;140(11):e596-646.
3. Mach F, Baigent C, Catapano AL, Koskinas KC, Casula M, Badimon L, et al. 2019 ESC/EAS guidelines for the management of dyslipidaemias: lipid modification to reduce cardiovascular risk. Eur Heart J. 2020;41(1):111–88.
4. McEvoy JW, Diamond GA, Detrano RC, Kaul S, Blaha MJ, Blumenthal RS, et al. Risk and the physics of clinical prediction. Am J Cardiol. 2014;113(8):1429–35.

5. Pender A, Lloyd-Jones DM, Stone NJ, Greenland P. Refining statin prescribing in lower-risk individuals: informing risk/benefit decisions. J Am Coll Cardiol. 2016;68(15):1690–7.

6. Amin NP, Martin SS, Blaha MJ, Nasir K, Blumenthal RS, Michos ED. Headed in the right direction but at risk for miscalculation: a critical appraisal of the 2013 ACC/AHA risk assessment guidelines. J Am College Cardiol. 2014;63(25 Pt A):2789–94.

7. Biomarkers and surrogate endpoints. Preferred definitions and conceptual framework. Clin Pharmacol Ther. 2001;69(3):89–95.

8. Vasan RS. Biomarkers of cardiovascular disease: molecular basis and practical considerations. Circulation. 2006;113(19):2335–62.

9. Osibogun O, Ogunmoroti O, Tibuakuu M, Benson EM, Michos ED. Sex differences in the association between ideal cardiovascular health and biomarkers of cardiovascular disease among adults in the United States: a cross-sectional analysis from the multiethnic study of atherosclerosis. BMJ Open. 2019;9(11):e031414.

10. Morrow DA, de Lemos JA. Benchmarks for the assessment of novel cardiovascular biomarkers. Circulation. 2007;115(8):949–52.

11. Kannel WB, Dawber TR, Kagan A, Revotskie N, Stokes J, 3rd. Factors of risk in the development of coronary heart disease–six year follow-up experience. The Framingham Study. Annals Internal Med. 1961;55:33–50.

12. Cholesterol Treatment Trialists C, Baigent C, Blackwell L, Emberson J, Holland LE, Reith C, et al. Efficacy and safety of more intensive lowering of LDL cholesterol: a meta-analysis of data from 170,000 participants in 26 randomised trials. Lancet (London, England). 2010;376(9753):1670–81.

13. Cholesterol Treatment Trialists C, Mihaylova B, Emberson J, Blackwell L, Keech A, Simes J, et al. The effects of lowering LDL cholesterol with statin therapy in people at low risk of vascular disease: meta-analysis of individual data from 27 randomised trials. Lancet (London, England). 2012;380(9841):581–90.

14. Ference BA, Ginsberg HN, Graham I, Ray KK, Packard CJ, Bruckert E, et al. Low-density lipoproteins cause atherosclerotic cardiovascular disease. 1. Evidence from genetic, epidemiologic, and clinical studies. A consensus statement from the European Atherosclerosis Society Consensus Panel. Eur Heart J. 2017;38(32):2459–72.

15. Michos ED, McEvoy JW, Blumenthal RS. Lipid management for the prevention of atherosclerotic cardiovascular disease. New England J Med. 2019;381(16):1557–67.

16. Castelli WP. Lipids, risk factors and ischaemic heart disease. Atherosclerosis. 1996;124 (Suppl):S1-9.

17. Sabatine MS, Wiviott SD, Im K, Murphy SA, Giugliano RP. Efficacy and safety of further lowering of low-density lipoprotein cholesterol in patients starting with very low levels: a meta-analysis. JAMA Cardiol. 2018;3(9):823–8.

18. Friedewald WT, Levy RI, Fredrickson DS. Estimation of the concentration of low-density lipoprotein cholesterol in plasma, without use of the preparative ultracentrifuge. Clin Chem. 1972;18(6):499–502.

19. Quispe R, Hendrani A, Elshazly MB, Michos ED, McEvoy JW, Blaha MJ, et al. Accuracy of low-density lipoprotein cholesterol estimation at very low levels. BMC Med. 2017;15(1):83.

20. Martin SS, Blaha MJ, Elshazly MB, Toth PP, Kwiterovich PO, Blumenthal RS, et al. Comparison of a novel method vs the friedewald equation for estimating low-density lipoprotein cholesterol levels from the standard lipid profile. JAMA. 2013;310(19):2061–8.

21. Pallazola VA, Sathiyakumar V, Ogunmoroti O, Fashanu O, Jones SR, Santos RD, et al. Impact of improved low-density lipoprotein cholesterol assessment on guideline classification in the modern treatment era-Results from a racially diverse Brazilian cross-sectional study. J Clin Lipidol. 2019;13(5):804–11 e2.

22. Chaen H, Kinchiku S, Miyata M, Kajiya S, Uenomachi H, Yuasa T, et al. Validity of a novel method for estimation of low-density lipoprotein cholesterol levels in diabetic patients. J Atheroscler Thromb. 2016;23(12):1355–64.

23. Lee J, Jang S, Son H. Validation of the Martin Method for Estimating Low-Density Lipoprotein Cholesterol Levels in Korean Adults: Findings from the Korea National Health and Nutrition Examination Survey, 2009–2011. PloS one. 2016;11(1):e0148147.

24. Mehta R, Reyes-Rodriguez E, Yaxmehen Bello-Chavolla O, Guerrero-Diaz AC, Vargas-Vazquez A, Cruz-Bautista I, et al. Performance of LDL-C calculated with Martin's formula compared to the Friedewald equation in familial combined hyperlipidemia. Atherosclerosis. 2018;277:204–10.

25. Martin SS, Giugliano RP, Murphy SA, Wasserman SM, Stein EA, Ceska R, et al. Comparison of low-density lipoprotein cholesterol assessment by martin/hopkins estimation, friedewald estimation, and preparative ultracentrifugation: insights from the FOURIER trial. JAMA Cardiol. 2018;3(8):749–53.

26. Khan SU, Khan MU, Valavoor S, Khan MS, Okunrintemi V, Mamas MA, et al. Association of lowering apolipoprotein B with cardiovascular outcomes across various lipid-lowering therapies: Systematic review and meta-analysis of trials. Eur J Prev Cardiol. 2019:2047487319871733.

27. Martin SS, Michos ED. Are we moving towards concordance on the principle that lipid discordance matters? Circulation. 2014;129(5):539–41.

28. Cromwell WC, Otvos JD, Keyes MJ, Pencina MJ, Sullivan L, Vasan RS, et al. LDL particle number and risk of future cardiovascular disease in the framingham offspring study—implications for LDL management. J Clin Lipidol. 2007;1(6):583–92.

29. Otvos JD, Mora S, Shalaurova I, Greenland P, Mackey RH, Goff DC Jr. Clinical implications of discordance between low-density lipoprotein cholesterol and particle number. J Clin Lipidol. 2011;5(2):105–13.

30. Mora S, Buring JE, Ridker PM. Discordance of low-density lipoprotein (LDL) cholesterol with alternative LDL-related measures and future coronary events. Circulation. 2014;129 (5):553–61.

31. Sniderman AD, St-Pierre AC, Cantin B, Dagenais GR, Despres JP, Lamarche B. Concordance/discordance between plasma apolipoprotein B levels and the cholesterol indexes of atherosclerotic risk. Am J Cardiol. 2003;91(10):1173–7.

32. Sniderman AD, Pencina M, Thanassoulis G. ApoB. Circ Res. 2019;124(10):1425–7.

33. Soedamah-Muthu SS, Chang YF, Otvos J, Evans RW, Orchard TJ, Pittsburgh Epidemiology of Diabetes Complications S. Lipoprotein subclass measurements by nuclear magnetic resonance spectroscopy improve the prediction of coronary artery disease in Type 1 diabetes. A prospective report from the Pittsburgh Epidemiology of Diabetes Complications Study. Diabetologia. 2003;46(5):674–82.

34. Sniderman AD, Williams K, McQueen MJ, Furberg CD. When is equal not equal? J Clin Lipidol. 2010;4(2):83–8.

35. Sniderman AD. Differential response of cholesterol and particle measures of atherogenic lipoproteins to LDL-lowering therapy: implications for clinical practice. J Clin Lipidol. 2008;2(1):36–42.

36. Sniderman AD, Islam S, Yusuf S, McQueen MJ. Discordance analysis of apolipoprotein B and non-high density lipoprotein cholesterol as markers of cardiovascular risk in the INTERHEART study. Atherosclerosis. 2012;225(2):444–9.

37. Emerging Risk Factors C, Di Angelantonio E, Sarwar N, Perry P, Kaptoge S, Ray KK, et al. Major lipids, apolipoproteins, and risk of vascular disease. JAMA. 2009;302(18):1993–2000.

38. Barter PJ, Ballantyne CM, Carmena R, Castro Cabezas M, Chapman MJ, Couture P, et al. Apo B versus cholesterol in estimating cardiovascular risk and in guiding therapy: report of the thirty-person/ten-country panel. J Intern Med. 2006;259(3):247–58.

39. Castelli WP. Cholesterol and lipids in the risk of coronary artery disease–the Framingham Heart Study. Can J Cardiol. 1988;4 Suppl A:5A-10A.

40. McQueen MJ, Hawken S, Wang X, Ounpuu S, Sniderman A, Probstfield J, et al. Lipids, lipoproteins, and apolipoproteins as risk markers of myocardial infarction in 52 countries

(the INTERHEART study): a case-control study. Lancet (London, England). 2008;372 (9634):224–33.

41. Ridker PM, Rifai N, Cook NR, Bradwin G, Buring JE. Non-HDL cholesterol, apolipoproteins A-I and B100, standard lipid measures, lipid ratios, and CRP as risk factors for cardiovascular disease in women. JAMA. 2005;294(3):326–33.

42. Mora S, Otvos JD, Rifai N, Rosenson RS, Buring JE, Ridker PM. Lipoprotein particle profiles by nuclear magnetic resonance compared with standard lipids and apolipoproteins in predicting incident cardiovascular disease in women. Circulation. 2009;119(7):931–9.

43. Prospective Studies C, Lewington S, Whitlock G, Clarke R, Sherliker P, Emberson J, et al. Blood cholesterol and vascular mortality by age, sex, and blood pressure: a meta-analysis of individual data from 61 prospective studies with 55,000 vascular deaths. Lancet (London, England). 2007;370(9602):1829–39.

44. Elshazly MB, Quispe R, Michos ED, Sniderman AD, Toth PP, Banach M, et al. Patient-level discordance in population percentiles of the total cholesterol to high-density lipoprotein cholesterol ratio in comparison with low-density lipoprotein cholesterol and non-high-density lipoprotein cholesterol: the very large database of lipids study (VLDL-2B). Circulation. 2015;132(8):667–76.

45. Elshazly MB, Nicholls SJ, Nissen SE, St John J, Martin SS, Jones SR, et al. Implications of total to high-density lipoprotein cholesterol ratio discordance with alternative lipid parameters for coronary atheroma progression and cardiovascular events. Am J Cardiol. 2016;118(5):647–55.

46. Quispe R, Elshazly MB, Zhao D, Toth PP, Puri R, Virani SS, et al. Total cholesterol/ HDL-cholesterol ratio discordance with LDL-cholesterol and non-HDL-cholesterol and incidence of atherosclerotic cardiovascular disease in primary prevention: The ARIC study. Eur J Prev Cardiol. 2019:2047487319862401.

47. Mathews SC, Mallidi J, Kulkarni K, Toth PP, Jones SR. Achieving secondary prevention low-density lipoprotein particle concentration goals using lipoprotein cholesterol-based data. PloS one. 2012;7(3):e33692.

48. Gardner CD, Fortmann SP, Krauss RM. Association of small low-density lipoprotein particles with the incidence of coronary artery disease in men and women. JAMA. 1996;276 (11):875–81.

49. Holmes MV, Asselbergs FW, Palmer TM, Drenos F, Lanktree MB, Nelson CP, et al. Mendelian randomization of blood lipids for coronary heart disease. Eur Heart J. 2015;36 (9):539–50.

50. Miller M, Stone NJ, Ballantyne C, Bittner V, Criqui MH, Ginsberg HN, et al. Triglycerides and cardiovascular disease: a scientific statement from the American heart association. Circulation. 2011;123(20):2292–333.

51. Schwartz GG, Olsson AG, Ezekowitz MD, Ganz P, Oliver MF, Waters D, et al. Effects of atorvastatin on early recurrent ischemic events in acute coronary syndromes: the MIRACL study: a randomized controlled trial. JAMA. 2001;285(13):1711–8.

52. Schwartz GG, Olsson AG, Abt M, Ballantyne CM, Barter PJ, Brumm J, et al. Effects of dalcetrapib in patients with a recent acute coronary syndrome. New England J Med. 2012;367(22):2089–99.

53. Schwartz GG, Abt M, Bao W, DeMicco D, Kallend D, Miller M, et al. Fasting triglycerides predict recurrent ischemic events in patients with acute coronary syndrome treated with statins. J Am Coll Cardiol. 2015;65(21):2267–75.

54. Miller M, Cannon CP, Murphy SA, Qin J, Ray KK, Braunwald E, et al. Impact of triglyceride levels beyond low-density lipoprotein cholesterol after acute coronary syndrome in the PROVE IT-TIMI 22 trial. J Am Coll Cardiol. 2008;51(7):724–30.

55. Bhatt DL, Steg PG, Miller M, Brinton EA, Jacobson TA, Ketchum SB, et al. Cardiovascular risk reduction with Icosapent Ethyl for Hypertriglyceridemia. New England J Med. 2019;380(1):11–22.

56. Group AS, Ginsberg HN, Elam MB, Lovato LC, Crouse JR, 3rd, Leiter LA, et al. Effects of combination lipid therapy in type 2 diabetes mellitus. New England J Med. 2010;362 (17):1563–74.

57. Guyton JR, Slee AE, Anderson T, Fleg JL, Goldberg RB, Kashyap ML, et al. Relationship of lipoproteins to cardiovascular events: the AIM-HIGH Trial (Atherothrombosis Intervention in Metabolic Syndrome With Low HDL/High Triglycerides and Impact on Global Health Outcomes). J Am Coll Cardiol. 2013;62(17):1580–4.

58. Nicholls SJ, Lincoff AM, Garcia M, Bash D, Ballantyne CM, Barter PJ, et al. Effect of high-dose omega-3 fatty acids vs corn oil on major adverse cardiovascular events in patients at high cardiovascular risk: the STRENGTH randomized clinical trial. JAMA. 2020;324 (22):2268–80.

59. Gaudet D, Alexander VJ, Baker BF, Brisson D, Tremblay K, Singleton W, et al. Antisense inhibition of apolipoprotein C-III in patients with hypertriglyceridemia. New England J Med. 2015;373(5):438–47.

60. Jorgensen AB, Frikke-Schmidt R, West AS, Grande P, Nordestgaard BG, Tybjaerg-Hansen A. Genetically elevated non-fasting triglycerides and calculated remnant cholesterol as causal risk factors for myocardial infarction. Eur Heart J. 2013;34(24):1826–33.

61. Varbo A, Benn M, Tybjaerg-Hansen A, Jorgensen AB, Frikke-Schmidt R, Nordestgaard BG. Remnant cholesterol as a causal risk factor for ischemic heart disease. J Am Coll Cardiol. 2013;61(4):427–36.

62. Jorgensen AB, Frikke-Schmidt R, Nordestgaard BG, Tybjaerg-Hansen A. Loss-of-function mutations in APOC3 and risk of ischemic vascular disease. New England J Med. 2014;371 (1):32–41.

63. Crosby J, Peloso GM, Auer PL, Crosslin DR, Stitziel NO, Lange LA, et al. Loss-of-function mutations in APOC3, triglycerides, and coronary disease. New England J Med. 2014;371 (1):22–31.

64. Elshazly MB, Mani P, Nissen S, Brennan DM, Clark D, Martin S, et al. Remnant cholesterol, coronary atheroma progression and clinical events in statin-treated patients with coronary artery disease. Eur J Prev Cardiol. 2019:2047487319887578.

65. Varbo A, Nordestgaard BG. Remnant lipoproteins. Curr Opin Lipidol. 2017;28(4):300–7.

66. Faridi KF, Quispe R, Martin SS, Hendrani AD, Joshi PH, Brinton EA, et al. Comparing different assessments of remnant lipoprotein cholesterol: the very large database of lipids. J Clin Lipidol. 2019;13(4):634–44.

67. Spence JD, Koschinsky M. Mechanisms of lipoprotein(a) pathogenicity: prothrombotic, proatherosclerotic, or both? Arterioscler Thromb Vasc Biol. 2012;32(7):1550–1.

68. Kamstrup PR, Tybjaerg-Hansen A, Steffensen R, Nordestgaard BG. Genetically elevated lipoprotein(a) and increased risk of myocardial infarction. JAMA. 2009;301(22):2331–9.

69. Nordestgaard BG, Langsted A. Lipoprotein (a) as a cause of cardiovascular disease: insights from epidemiology, genetics, and biology. J Lipid Res. 2016;57(11):1953–75.

70. Emerging Risk Factors C, Erqou S, Kaptoge S, Perry PL, Di Angelantonio E, Thompson A, et al. Lipoprotein(a) concentration and the risk of coronary heart disease, stroke, and nonvascular mortality. Jama. 2009;302(4):412–23.

71. Pare G, Caku A, McQueen M, Anand SS, Enas E, Clarke R, et al. Lipoprotein(a) levels and the risk of myocardial infarction among 7 ethnic groups. Circulation. 2019;139(12):1472–82.

72. O'Donoghue ML, Fazio S, Giugliano RP, Stroes ESG, Kanevsky E, Gouni-Berthold I, et al. Lipoprotein(a), PCSK9 inhibition, and cardiovascular risk. Circulation. 2019;139(12):1483–92.

73. Tsimikas S, Karwatowska-Prokopczuk E, Gouni-Berthold I, Tardif JC, Baum SJ, Steinhagen-Thiessen E, et al. Lipoprotein(a) reduction in persons with cardiovascular disease. New England J Med. 2020;382(3):244–55.

74. Tsimikas S. A test in context: lipoprotein(a): diagnosis, prognosis, controversies, and emerging therapies. J Am Coll Cardiol. 2017;69(6):692–711.

75. Albers JJ, Slee A, O'Brien KD, Robinson JG, Kashyap ML, Kwiterovich PO Jr, et al. Relationship of apolipoproteins A-1 and B, and lipoprotein(a) to cardiovascular outcomes: the AIM-HIGH trial (Atherothrombosis Intervention in Metabolic Syndrome with Low

HDL/High Triglyceride and Impact on Global Health Outcomes). J Am Coll Cardiol. 2013;62(17):1575–9.

76. Willeit P, Kiechl S, Kronenberg F, Witztum JL, Santer P, Mayr M, et al. Discrimination and net reclassification of cardiovascular risk with lipoprotein(a): prospective 15-year outcomes in the Bruneck Study. J Am Coll Cardiol. 2014;64(9):851–60.

77. Verbeek R, Sandhu MS, Hovingh GK, Sjouke B, Wareham NJ, Zwinderman AH, et al. Lipoprotein(a) improves cardiovascular risk prediction based on established risk algorithms. J Am Coll Cardiol. 2017;69(11):1513–5.

78. Kamstrup PR, Tybjaerg-Hansen A, Nordestgaard BG. Extreme lipoprotein(a) levels and improved cardiovascular risk prediction. J Am Coll Cardiol. 2013;61(11):1146–56.

79. Fogacci F, Cicero AF, D'Addato S, D'Agostini L, Rosticci M, Giovannini M, et al. Serum lipoprotein(a) level as long-term predictor of cardiovascular mortality in a large sample of subjects in primary cardiovascular prevention: data from the Brisighella heart study. Eur J Intern Med. 2017;37:49–55.

80. Xie H, Chen L, Liu H, Cui Y, Zhang Z, Cui L. Long-term prognostic value of lipoprotein(a) in symptomatic patients with nonobstructive coronary artery disease. Am J Cardiol. 2017;119(7):945–50.

81. Suwa S, Ogita M, Miyauchi K, Sonoda T, Konishi H, Tsuboi S, et al. Impact of lipoprotein (a) on long-term outcomes in patients with coronary artery disease treated with statin after a first percutaneous coronary intervention. J Atheroscler Thromb. 2017;24(11):1125–31.

82. Boden WE, Sidhu MS, Toth PP. The therapeutic role of niacin in dyslipidemia management. J Cardiovasc Pharmacol Ther. 2014;19(2):141–58.

83. Burgess S, Ference BA, Staley JR, Freitag DF, Mason AM, Nielsen SF, et al. Association of LPA variants with risk of coronary disease and the implications for lipoprotein(a)-lowering therapies: a mendelian randomization analysis. JAMA Cardiol. 2018;3(7):619–27.

84. Wilson DP, Jacobson TA, Jones PH, Koschinsky ML, McNeal CJ, Nordestgaard BG, et al. Use of Lipoprotein(a) in clinical practice: a biomarker whose time has come. A scientific statement from the National Lipid Association. J Clin Lipidol. 2019;13(3):374–92.

85. Sharma S, Jackson PG, Makan J. Cardiac troponins. J Clin Pathol. 2004;57(10):1025–6.

86. Apple FS, Collinson PO, Biomarkers ITFoCAoC. Analytical characteristics of high-sensitivity cardiac troponin assays. Clin Chem. 2012;58(1):54–61.

87. Iwanaga Y, Nishi I, Furuichi S, Noguchi T, Sase K, Kihara Y, et al. B-type natriuretic peptide strongly reflects diastolic wall stress in patients with chronic heart failure: comparison between systolic and diastolic heart failure. J Am Coll Cardiol. 2006;47(4):742–8.

88. Brunner-La Rocca HP, Kaye DM, Woods RL, Hastings J, Esler MD. Effects of intravenous brain natriuretic peptide on regional sympathetic activity in patients with chronic heart failure as compared with healthy control subjects. J Am Coll Cardiol. 2001;37(5):1221–7.

89. Michos ED, Wilson LM, Yeh HC, Berger Z, Suarez-Cuervo C, Stacy SR, et al. Prognostic value of cardiac troponin in patients with chronic kidney disease without suspected acute coronary syndrome: a systematic review and meta-analysis. Ann Intern Med. 2014;161 (7):491–501.

90. McCullough PA, Duc P, Omland T, McCord J, Nowak RM, Hollander JE, et al. B-type natriuretic peptide and renal function in the diagnosis of heart failure: an analysis from the breathing not properly multinational study. Am J Kidney Dis. 2003;41(3):571–9.

91. Ying W, Zhao D, Ouyang P, Subramanya V, Vaidya D, Ndumele CE, et al. Sex hormones and change in N-terminal Pro-B-type natriuretic peptide levels: the multi-ethnic study of atherosclerosis. J Clin Endocrinol Metabol. 2018;103(11):4304–14.

92. Gore MO, Seliger SL, Defilippi CR, Nambi V, Christenson RH, Hashim IA, et al. Age- and sex-dependent upper reference limits for the high-sensitivity cardiac troponin T assay. J Am Coll Cardiol. 2014;63(14):1441–8.

93. Lee KK, Ferry AV, Anand A, Strachan FE, Chapman AR, Kimenai DM, et al. Sex-specific thresholds of high-sensitivity troponin in patients with suspected acute coronary syndrome. J Am Coll Cardiol. 2019;74(16):2032–43.

94. Keyzer JM, Hoffmann JJ, Ringoir L, Nabbe KC, Widdershoven JW, Pop VJ. Age- and gender-specific brain natriuretic peptide (BNP) reference ranges in primary care. Clin Chem Lab Med. 2014;52(9):1341–6.

95. Sherwood MW, Kristin Newby L. High-sensitivity troponin assays: evidence, indications, and reasonable use. J Am Heart Assoc. 2014;3(1):e000403.

96. Tate JR, Bunk DM, Christenson RH, Katrukha A, Noble JE, Porter RA, et al. Standardisation of cardiac troponin I measurement: past and present. Pathology. 2010;42 (5):402–8.

97. Clerico A, Zaninotto M, Prontera C, Giovannini S, Ndreu R, Franzini M, et al. State of the art of BNP and NT-proBNP immunoassays: the CardioOrmoCheck study. Clin Chim Acta; Int J Clin Chem. 2012;414:112–9.

98. de Lemos JA, Drazner MH, Omland T, Ayers CR, Khera A, Rohatgi A, et al. Association of troponin T detected with a highly sensitive assay and cardiac structure and mortality risk in the general population. JAMA. 2010;304(22):2503–12.

99. Martin Raymondi D, Garcia H, Alvarez I, Hernandez L, Molinero JP, Villamandos V. TUSARC: prognostic value of high-sensitivity cardiac troponin T assay in asymptomatic patients with high cardiovascular risk. Am J Med. 2019;132(5):631–8.

100. Ford I, Shah AS, Zhang R, McAllister DA, Strachan FE, Caslake M, et al. High-sensitivity cardiac troponin, statin therapy, and risk of coronary heart disease. J Am Coll Cardiol. 2016;68(25):2719–28.

101. Jia X, Sun W, Hoogeveen RC, Nambi V, Matsushita K, Folsom AR, et al. High-sensitivity troponin i and incident coronary events, stroke, heart failure hospitalization, and mortality in the ARIC study. Circulation. 2019;139(23):2642–53.

102. Lan NSR, Bell DA, McCaul KA, Vasikaran SD, Yeap BB, Norman PE, et al. High-sensitivity cardiac troponin i improves cardiovascular risk prediction in older men: HIMS (The Health in Men Study). J Am Heart Assoc. 2019;8(5):e011818.

103. McEvoy JW, Chen Y, Nambi V, Ballantyne CM, Sharrett AR, Appel LJ, et al. High-sensitivity cardiac troponin T and risk of hypertension. Circulation. 2015;132 (9):825–33.

104. Pandey A, Patel KV, Vongpatanasin W, Ayers C, Berry JD, Mentz RJ, et al. Incorporation of biomarkers into risk assessment for allocation of antihypertensive medication according to the 2017 ACC/AHA high blood pressure guideline: a pooled cohort analysis. Circulation. 2019;140(25):2076–88.

105. Kang DH, Park SJ, Lee SA, Lee S, Kim DH, Kim HK, et al. Early surgery or conservative care for asymptomatic aortic stenosis. New England J Med. 2020;382(2):111–9.

106. Baumgartner H, Falk V, Bax JJ, De Bonis M, Hamm C, Holm PJ, et al. 2017 ESC/EACTS guidelines for the management of valvular heart disease. Eur Heart J. 2017;38(36):2739–91.

107. McCarthy CP, Donnellan E, Phelan D, Griffin BP, Enriquez-Sarano M, McEvoy JW. High sensitivity troponin and valvular heart disease. Trends Cardiovasc Med. 2017;27(5):326–33.

108. Chin CW, Shah AS, McAllister DA, Joanna Cowell S, Alam S, Langrish JP, et al. High-sensitivity troponin I concentrations are a marker of an advanced hypertrophic response and adverse outcomes in patients with aortic stenosis. Eur Heart J. 2014;35 (34):2312–21.

109. Ferrer-Sistach E, Lupon J, Cediel G, Teis A, Gual F, Serrano S, et al. High-sensitivity troponin T in asymptomatic severe aortic stenosis. Biomarkers. 2019;24(4):334–40.

110. Chin CW, Messika-Zeitoun D, Shah AS, Lefevre G, Bailleul S, Yeung EN, et al. A clinical risk score of myocardial fibrosis predicts adverse outcomes in aortic stenosis. Eur Heart J. 2016;37(8):713–23.

111. Velagaleti RS, Gona P, Larson MG, Wang TJ, Levy D, Benjamin EJ, et al. Multimarker approach for the prediction of heart failure incidence in the community. Circulation. 2010;122(17):1700–6.

112. Saunders JT, Nambi V, de Lemos JA, Chambless LE, Virani SS, Boerwinkle E, et al. Cardiac troponin T measured by a highly sensitive assay predicts coronary heart disease,

heart failure, and mortality in the atherosclerosis risk in communities study. Circulation. 2011;123(13):1367–76.

113. Ledwidge M, Gallagher J, Conlon C, Tallon E, O'Connell E, Dawkins I, et al. Natriuretic peptide-based screening and collaborative care for heart failure: the STOP-HF randomized trial. JAMA. 2013;310(1):66–74.

114. McGrady M, Reid CM, Shiel L, Wolfe R, Boffa U, Liew D, et al. NT-proB natriuretic peptide, risk factors and asymptomatic left ventricular dysfunction: results of the SCReening evaluation of the evolution of new heart failure study (SCREEN-HF). Int J Cardiol. 2013;169(2):133–8.

115. Chow SL, Maisel AS, Anand I, Bozkurt B, de Boer RA, Felker GM, et al. Role of biomarkers for the prevention, assessment, and management of heart failure: a scientific statement from the american heart association. Circulation. 2017;135(22):e1054–91.

116. Libby P. Interleukin-1 beta as a target for atherosclerosis therapy: biological basis of CANTOS and beyond. J Am Coll Cardiol. 2017;70(18):2278–89.

117. Esmon CT. Inflammation and thrombosis. J Thrombosis Haemostasis: JTH. 2003;1 (7):1343–8.

118. Ridker PM, Hennekens CH, Buring JE, Rifai N. C-reactive protein and other markers of inflammation in the prediction of cardiovascular disease in women. New England J Med. 2000;342(12):836–43.

119. Schonbeck U, Libby P. Inflammation, immunity, and HMG-CoA reductase inhibitors: statins as antiinflammatory agents? Circulation. 2004;109(21 Suppl 1):II18–26.

120. Labos C, Brophy JM, Smith GD, Sniderman AD, Thanassoulis G. Evaluation of the pleiotropic effects of statins: a reanalysis of the randomized trial evidence using egger regression-brief report. Arterioscler Thromb Vasc Biol. 2018;38(1):262–5.

121. Ridker PM, Danielson E, Fonseca FA, Genest J, Gotto AM Jr, Kastelein JJ, et al. Rosuvastatin to prevent vascular events in men and women with elevated C-reactive protein. N Engl J Med. 2008;359(21):2195–207.

122. Ridker PM, Everett BM, Thuren T, MacFadyen JG, Chang WH, Ballantyne C, et al. Antiinflammatory therapy with Canakinumab for atherosclerotic disease. New England J Med. 2017;377(12):1119–31.

123. Duprez DA, Otvos J, Sanchez OA, Mackey RH, Tracy R, Jacobs DR Jr. Comparison of the predictive value of GlycA and other biomarkers of inflammation for total death, incident cardiovascular events, noncardiovascular and noncancer inflammatory-related events, and total cancer events. Clin Chem. 2016;62(7):1020–31.

124. Quispe R, Michos ED, Martin SS, Puri R, Toth PP, Al Suwaidi J, et al. High-sensitivity C-reactive protein discordance with atherogenic lipid measures and incidence of atherosclerotic cardiovascular disease in primary prevention: the ARIC study. J Am Heart Assoc. 2020;9(3):e013600.

125. Ridker PM, Buring JE, Rifai N, Cook NR. Development and validation of improved algorithms for the assessment of global cardiovascular risk in women: the Reynolds Risk Score. JAMA. 2007;297(6):611–9.

126. Ridker PM, Paynter NP, Rifai N, Gaziano JM, Cook NR. C-reactive protein and parental history improve global cardiovascular risk prediction: the Reynolds Risk Score for men. Circulation. 2008;118(22):2243–51, 4p following 51.

127. Michos ED, Martin SS, Blumenthal RS. Bringing back targets to "IMPROVE" atherosclerotic cardiovascular disease outcomes: the duel for dual goals; are two targets better than one? Circulation. 2015;132(13):1218–20.

128. Michos ED, Blumenthal RS. Treatment concentration of high-sensitivity C-reactive protein. Lancet (London, England). 2018;391(10118):287–9.

129. Cardoso R, Kaul S, Okada DR, Blumenthal RS, Michos ED. A deeper dive into the CANTOS "Responders" Substudy. Mayo Clin Proc. 2018;93(7):830–3.

130. Ridker PM, Danielson E, Fonseca FA, Genest J, Gotto AM Jr, Kastelein JJ, et al. Reduction in C-reactive protein and LDL cholesterol and cardiovascular event rates after initiation of

rosuvastatin: a prospective study of the JUPITER trial. Lancet (London, England). 2009;373 (9670):1175–82.

131. Ridker PM, Morrow DA, Rose LM, Rifai N, Cannon CP, Braunwald E. Relative efficacy of atorvastatin 80 mg and pravastatin 40 mg in achieving the dual goals of low-density lipoprotein cholesterol <70 mg/dl and C-reactive protein <2 mg/l: an analysis of the PROVE-IT TIMI-22 trial. J Am Coll Cardiol. 2005;45(10):1644–8.

132. Bohula EA, Giugliano RP, Cannon CP, Zhou J, Murphy SA, White JA, et al. Achievement of dual low-density lipoprotein cholesterol and high-sensitivity C-reactive protein targets more frequent with the addition of ezetimibe to simvastatin and associated with better outcomes in IMPROVE-IT. Circulation. 2015;132(13):1224–33.

133. Ridker PM, MacFadyen JG, Everett BM, Libby P, Thuren T, Glynn RJ, et al. Relationship of C-reactive protein reduction to cardiovascular event reduction following treatment with canakinumab: a secondary analysis from the CANTOS randomised controlled trial. Lancet (London, England). 2018;391(10118):319–28.

134. Otvos JD, Shalaurova I, Wolak-Dinsmore J, Connelly MA, Mackey RH, Stein JH, et al. GlycA: a composite nuclear magnetic resonance biomarker of systemic inflammation. Clin Chem. 2015;61(5):714–23.

135. Akinkuolie AO, Buring JE, Ridker PM, Mora S. A novel protein glycan biomarker and future cardiovascular disease events. J Am Heart Assoc. 2014;3(5):e001221.

136. Akinkuolie AO, Glynn RJ, Padmanabhan L, Ridker PM, Mora S. Circulating N-linked glycoprotein side-Chain biomarker, rosuvastatin therapy, and incident cardiovascular disease: an analysis from the JUPITER trial. J Am Heart Assoc. 2016;5(7).

137. Fashanu OE, Oyenuga AO, Zhao D, Tibuakuu M, Mora S, Otvos JD, et al. GlycA, a novel inflammatory marker and its association with peripheral arterial disease and carotid plaque: the multi-ethnic study of atherosclerosis. Angiology. 2019;70(8):737–46.

138. Gruppen EG, Riphagen IJ, Connelly MA, Otvos JD, Bakker SJ, Dullaart RP. GlycA, a Pro-inflammatory glycoprotein biomarker, and incident cardiovascular disease: relationship with C-reactive protein and renal function. PloS one. 2015;10(9):e0139057.

139. Lawler PR, Akinkuolie AO, Chandler PD, Moorthy MV, Vandenburgh MJ, Schaumberg DA, et al. Circulating N-linked glycoprotein acetyls and longitudinal mortality risk. Circ Res. 2016;118(7):1106–15.

140. Jang S, Ogunmoroti O, Ndumele CE, Zhao D, Rao VN, Fashanu OE, et al. Association of the novel inflammatory marker GlycA and incident heart failure and its subtypes of preserved and reduced ejection fraction: the multi-ethnic study of atherosclerosis. Circ Heart Fail. 2020;13(8):e007067.

141. Benson EA, Tibuakuu M, Zhao D, Akinkuolie AO, Otvos JD, Duprez DA, et al. Associations of ideal cardiovascular health with GlycA, a novel inflammatory marker: the Multi-Ethnic Study of Atherosclerosis. Clin Cardiol. 2018;41(11):1439–45.

142. Tibuakuu M, Fashanu OE, Zhao D, Otvos JD, Brown TT, Haberlen SA, et al. GlycA, a novel inflammatory marker, is associated with subclinical coronary disease. AIDS. 2019;33 (3):547–57.

143. Joshi AA, Lerman JB, Aberra TM, Afshar M, Teague HL, Rodante JA, et al. GlycA is a novel biomarker of inflammation and subclinical cardiovascular disease in psoriasis. Circ Res. 2016;119(11):1242–53.

144. Ezeigwe A, Fashanu OE, Zhao D, Budoff MJ, Otvos JD, Thomas IC, et al. The novel inflammatory marker GlycA and the prevalence and progression of valvular and thoracic aortic calcification: the Multi-Ethnic Study of Atherosclerosis. Atherosclerosis. 2019;282:91–9.

145. Knight B, Xue Y, Maisel AS, de Boer RA. Galectin 3: newest marker of HF outcomes. Curr Emerg Hosp Med Rep. 2014;2(2):112–9.

146. Yu L, Ruifrok WP, Meissner M, Bos EM, van Goor H, Sanjabi B, et al. Genetic and pharmacological inhibition of galectin-3 prevents cardiac remodeling by interfering with myocardial fibrogenesis. Circ Heart Fail. 2013;6(1):107–17.

147. de Boer RA, van Veldhuisen DJ, Gansevoort RT, Muller Kobold AC, van Gilst WH, Hillege HL, et al. The fibrosis marker galectin-3 and outcome in the general population. J Intern Med. 2012;272(1):55–64.
148. McEvoy JW, Chen Y, Halushka MK, Christenson E, Ballantyne CM, Blumenthal RS, et al. Galectin-3 and risk of heart failure and death in blacks and whites. J Am Heart Assoc. 2016;5(5).
149. Maiolino G, Bisogni V, Rossitto G, Rossi GP. Lipoprotein-associated phospholipase A2 prognostic role in atherosclerotic complications. World J Cardiol. 2015;7(10):609–20.
150. Ballantyne CM, Hoogeveen RC, Bang H, Coresh J, Folsom AR, Heiss G, et al. Lipoprotein-associated phospholipase A2, high-sensitivity C-reactive protein, and risk for incident coronary heart disease in middle-aged men and women in the Atherosclerosis Risk in Communities (ARIC) study. Circulation. 2004;109(7):837–42.
151. Tibuakuu M, Kianoush S, DeFilippis AP, McEvoy JW, Zhao D, Guallar E, et al. Usefulness of lipoprotein-associated phospholipase A2 activity and C-reactive protein in identifying high-risk smokers for atherosclerotic cardiovascular disease (from the Atherosclerosis Risk in Communities Study). Am J Cardiol. 2018;121(9):1056–64.
152. Ridker PM, MacFadyen JG, Wolfert RL, Koenig W. Relationship of lipoprotein-associated phospholipase A(2) mass and activity with incident vascular events among primary prevention patients allocated to placebo or to statin therapy: an analysis from the JUPITER trial. Clin Chem. 2012;58(5):877–86.
153. Davidson MH, Corson MA, Alberts MJ, Anderson JL, Gorelick PB, Jones PH, et al. Consensus panel recommendation for incorporating lipoprotein-associated phospholipase A2 testing into cardiovascular disease risk assessment guidelines. Am J Cardiol. 2008;101 (12A):51F-F57.
154. Wang J, Tan GJ, Han LN, Bai YY, He M, Liu HB. Novel biomarkers for cardiovascular risk prediction. J Geriatr Cardiol. 2017;14(2):135–50.
155. Investigators S, White HD, Held C, Stewart R, Tarka E, Brown R, et al. Darapladib for preventing ischemic events in stable coronary heart disease. New England J Med. 2014;370 (18):1702–11.
156. Forte G, Minieri M, Cossa P, Antenucci D, Sala M, Gnocchi V, et al. Hepatocyte growth factor effects on mesenchymal stem cells: proliferation, migration, and differentiation. Stem Cells. 2006;24(1):23–33.
157. Rong S-l, Wang X-l, Wang Y-c, Wu H, Zhou X-d, Wang Z-k, et al. Anti-inflammatory activities of hepatocyte growth factor in post-ischemic heart failure. Acta Pharmacol Sinica. 2018;39(10):1613–21.
158. Bielinski SJ, Berardi C, Decker PA, Larson NB, Bell EJ, Pankow JS, et al. Hepatocyte growth factor demonstrates racial heterogeneity as a biomarker for coronary heart disease. Heart (British Cardiac Society). 2017;103(15):1185–93.
159. Morishita R, Aoki M, Yo Y, Ogihara T. Hepatocyte growth factor as cardiovascular hormone: role of HGF in the pathogenesis of cardiovascular disease. Endocr J. 2002;49 (3):273–84.
160. Rajpathak Swapnil N, Wang T, Wassertheil-Smoller S, Strickler Howard D, Kaplan Robert C, McGinn Aileen P, et al. Hepatocyte growth factor and the risk of ischemic stroke developing among postmenopausal women. Stroke. 2010;41(5):857–62.
161. Bell EJ, Larson NB, Decker PA, Pankow JS, Tsai MY, Hanson NQ, et al. Hepatocyte growth factor is positively associated with risk of stroke: the MESA (Multi-Ethnic Study of Atherosclerosis). Stroke. 2016;47(11):2689–94.
162. Decker PA, Larson NB, Bell EJ, Pankow JS, Hanson NQ, Wassel CL, et al. Increased hepatocyte growth factor levels over 2 years are associated with coronary heart disease: the Multi-Ethnic Study of Atherosclerosis (MESA). Am Heart J. 2019;213:30–4.
163. Bell EJ, Decker PA, Tsai MY, Pankow JS, Hanson NQ, Wassel CL, et al. Hepatocyte growth factor is associated with progression of atherosclerosis: the Multi-Ethnic Study of Atherosclerosis (MESA). Atherosclerosis. 2018;272:162–7.

164. Ferraro RA, Ogunmoroti O, Zhao D, Ndumele CE, Rao V, Pandey A, et al. Abstract 264: the association of hepatocyte growth factor with incident heart failure and its subtypes: the Multi-Ethnic Study of Atherosclerosis. Arterioscl. Thrombosis Vascul Biol. 2020;40 (Suppl_1):A264-A.

165. Ferraro RA, Ogunmoroti O, Zhao D, Ndumele CE, Lima JAC, Subramanya V, et al. Abstract 13300: hepatocyte growth factor and 10-year change in left ventricular structure: the Multi-Ethnic Study of Atherosclerosis. Circulation. 2020;142(Suppl_3):A13300-A.

166. Rychli K, Richter B, Hohensinner PJ, Mahdy Ali K, Neuhold S, Zorn G, et al. Hepatocyte growth factor is a strong predictor of mortality in patients with advanced heart failure. Heart. 2011;97(14):1158.

167. Bancks MP, Bielinski SJ, Decker PA, Hanson NQ, Larson NB, Sicotte H, et al. Circulating level of hepatocyte growth factor predicts incidence of type 2 diabetes mellitus: the Multi-Ethnic Study of Atherosclerosis (MESA). Metabolism. 2016;65(3):64–72.

168. Fibrinogen Studies C, Danesh J, Lewington S, Thompson SG, Lowe GD, Collins R, et al. Plasma fibrinogen level and the risk of major cardiovascular diseases and nonvascular mortality: an individual participant meta-analysis. JAMA. 2005;294(14):1799–809.

169. Perk J, De Backer G, Gohlke H, Graham I, Reiner Z, Verschuren M, et al. European guidelines on cardiovascular disease prevention in clinical practice (version 2012). The fifth joint task force of the European society of cardiology and other societies on cardiovascular disease prevention in clinical practice (constituted by representatives of nine societies and by invited experts). Eur Heart J. 2012;33(13):1635–701.

170. Piepoli MF, Hoes AW, Agewall S, Albus C, Brotons C, Catapano AL, et al. 2016 European guidelines on cardiovascular disease prevention in clinical practice: the sixth joint task force of the European society of cardiology and other societies on cardiovascular disease prevention in clinical practice (constituted by representatives of 10 societies and by invited experts) developed with the special contribution of the European Association for Cardiovascular Prevention & Rehabilitation (EACPR). Atherosclerosis. 2016;252:207–74.

171. Lau WB, Ohashi K, Wang Y, Ogawa H, Murohara T, Ma XL, et al. Role of adipokines in cardiovascular disease. Circ J. 2017;81(7):920–8.

172. Dutheil F, Gordon BA, Naughton G, Crendal E, Courteix D, Chaplais E, et al. Cardiovascular risk of adipokines: a review. J Int Med Res. 2018;46(6):2082–95.

173. Wannamethee SG, Lowe GD, Rumley A, Cherry L, Whincup PH, Sattar N. Adipokines and risk of type 2 diabetes in older men. Diabetes Care. 2007;30(5):1200–5.

174. Muse ED, Feldman DI, Blaha MJ, Dardari ZA, Blumenthal RS, Budoff MJ, et al. The association of resistin with cardiovascular disease in the Multi-Ethnic Study of Atherosclerosis. Atherosclerosis. 2015;239(1):101–8.

175. Pischon T, Girman CJ, Hotamisligil GS, Rifai N, Hu FB, Rimm EB. Plasma adiponectin levels and risk of myocardial infarction in men. JAMA. 2004;291(14):1730–7.

176. Landecho MF, Tuero C, Valenti V, Bilbao I, de la Higuera M, Fruhbeck G. Relevance of Leptin and other Adipokines in obesity-associated cardiovascular risk. Nutrients. 2019;11 (11).

177. Martin SS, Blaha MJ, Muse ED, Qasim AN, Reilly MP, Blumenthal RS, et al. Leptin and incident cardiovascular disease: the Multi-ethnic Study of Atherosclerosis (MESA). Atherosclerosis. 2015;239(1):67–72.

178. Fasshauer M, Bluher M, Stumvoll M. Adipokines in gestational diabetes. Lancet Diabetes Endocrinol. 2014;2(6):488–99.

179. Rodriguez CP, O. O, Quispe R, Osibogun OI, Ndumele CE, Echouffo Tcheugui JB, et al. Abstract 13525: The association between multiparity and Adipokine levels: the Multi-Ethnic Study of Atherosclerosis (MESA). Circulation. 2020;142(Suppl_3):A13525-A.

180. Jensen MK, Bertoia ML, Cahill LE, Agarwal I, Rimm EB, Mukamal KJ. Novel metabolic biomarkers of cardiovascular disease. Nat Rev Endocrinol. 2014;10(11):659–72.

181. Sattar N, Wannamethee G, Sarwar N, Tchernova J, Cherry L, Wallace AM, et al. Adiponectin and coronary heart disease: a prospective study and meta-analysis. Circulation. 2006;114(7):623–9.

182. Barouch LA, Berkowitz DE, Harrison RW, O'Donnell CP, Hare JM. Disruption of leptin signaling contributes to cardiac hypertrophy independently of body weight in mice. Circulation. 2003;108(6):754–9.
183. Ho JE, Lyass A, Courchesne P, Chen G, Liu C, Yin X, et al. Protein biomarkers of cardiovascular disease and mortality in the community. J Am Heart Assoc. 2018;7(14).
184. Acquarone E, Monacelli F, Borghi R, Nencioni A, Odetti P. Resistin: a reappraisal. Mech Ageing Dev. 2019;178:46–63.
185. Honigberg MC, Zekavat SM, Aragam K, Finneran P, Klarin D, Bhatt DL, et al. Association of premature natural and surgical menopause with incident cardiovascular disease. Jama. 2019.
186. Zhao D, Guallar E, Ouyang P, Subramanya V, Vaidya D, Ndumele CE, et al. Endogenous sex hormones and incident cardiovascular disease in post-menopausal women. J Am Coll Cardiol. 2018;71(22):2555–66.
187. Subramanya V, Zhao D, Ouyang P, Lima JA, Vaidya D, Ndumele CE, et al. Sex hormone levels and change in left ventricular structure among men and post-menopausal women: the Multi-Ethnic Study of Atherosclerosis (MESA). Maturitas. 2018;108:37–44.
188. Subramanya V, Ambale-Venkatesh B, Ohyama Y, Zhao D, Nwabuo CC, Post WS, et al. Relation of sex hormone levels with prevalent and 10-year change in aortic distensibility assessed by MRI: the multi-ethnic study of atherosclerosis. Am J Hypertens. 2018;31 (7):774–83.
189. Subramanya V, Zhao D, Ouyang P, Ying W, Vaidya D, Ndumele CE, et al. Association of endogenous sex hormone levels with coronary artery calcium progression among post-menopausal women in the Multi-Ethnic Study of Atherosclerosis (MESA). J Cardiovascul Comp Tomography. 2019;13(1):41–7.
190. Mathews L, Subramanya V, Zhao D, Ouyang P, Vaidya D, Guallar E, et al. Endogenous sex hormones and endothelial function in postmenopausal women and men: the multi-ethnic study of atherosclerosis. J Women's Health (2002). 2019;28(7):900–9.
191. Jia X, Sun C, Tang O, Gorlov I, Nambi V, Virani SS, et al. Plasma dehydroepiandrosterone sulfate and cardiovascular disease risk in older men and women. J Clin Endocrinol Metabol. 2020;105(12).
192. Akishita M, Hashimoto M, Ohike Y, Ogawa S, Iijima K, Eto M, et al. Low testosterone level as a predictor of cardiovascular events in Japanese men with coronary risk factors. Atherosclerosis. 2010;210(1):232–6.
193. Menke A, Guallar E, Rohrmann S, Nelson WG, Rifai N, Kanarek N, et al. Sex steroid hormone concentrations and risk of death in US men. Am J Epidemiol. 2010;171(5):583–92.
194. DeFilippis AP, Young R, McEvoy JW, Michos ED, Sandfort V, Kronmal RA, et al. Risk score overestimation: the impact of individual cardiovascular risk factors and preventive therapies on the performance of the American heart association-American college of cardiology-atherosclerotic cardiovascular disease risk score in a modern multi-ethnic cohort. Eur Heart J. 2017;38(8):598–608.
195. Yeboah J, McClelland RL, Polonsky TS, Burke GL, Sibley CT, O'Leary D, et al. Comparison of novel risk markers for improvement in cardiovascular risk assessment in intermediate-risk individuals. JAMA. 2012;308(8):788–95.
196. Yeboah J, Young R, McClelland RL, Delaney JC, Polonsky TS, Dawood FZ, et al. Utility of nontraditional risk markers in atherosclerotic cardiovascular disease risk assessment. J Am Coll Cardiol. 2016;67(2):139–47.
197. Blaha MJ, Cainzos-Achirica M, Greenland P, McEvoy JW, Blankstein R, Budoff MJ, et al. Role of coronary artery calcium score of zero and other negative risk markers for cardiovascular disease: the Multi-Ethnic Study of Atherosclerosis (MESA). Circulation. 2016;133(9):849–58.
198. Michos ED, Blaha MJ, Blumenthal RS. Use of the coronary artery calcium score in discussion of initiation of statin therapy in primary prevention. Mayo Clin Proc. 2017;92 (12):1831–41.

Genetics

Marios Arvanitis, Wendy S. Post, and Alexis Battle

Introduction

The discovery of next generation sequencing in the 1990s [1] along with the rapid rise in computing power over the past decade has led to an unprecedented broadening of our understanding of genetic processes that underlie disease biology. It is ever more appreciated that we are living in an era of a genomic revolution, one of enormous magnitude and scale, capable of reshaping our understanding of biological processes [2]. Indeed, the twenty-first century literature has seen an impressive rise in the number of publications regarding genomics [3].

Although this genomic analysis revolution has until recently been limited to research, it is increasingly understood that we are approaching a new phase in which genomic analyses will be translated into everyday clinical medicine [4]. Cardiovascular disease, being the primary cause of death worldwide and one of the most challenging public health concerns, has traditionally been at the forefront of changes in medical practice. For example, evidence-based medicine, which is considered a crucial aspect of current clinical practice, thrived within cardiology with multiple randomized trials dating back to the 1980s [5] before its official introduction as a term [6]. Therefore, it is not surprising to see the first signs of the integration of genomics into medicine within the field of Cardiovascular Disease Prevention.

M. Arvanitis · W. S. Post
Department of Medicine, Division of Cardiology, Johns Hopkins University,
Baltimore, MD, USA

M. Arvanitis · A. Battle (✉)
Department of Biomedical Engineering, Johns Hopkins University,
South Wing S349, 3100 Wyman Park Drive, Baltimore, MD 21211, USA
e-mail: ajbattle@jhu.edu

W. S. Post
Department of Epidemiology, Johns Hopkins Bloomberg School of Public Health,
Baltimore, MD, USA

© Springer Nature Switzerland AG 2021
S. S. Martin (ed.), *Precision Medicine in Cardiovascular Disease Prevention*,
https://doi.org/10.1007/978-3-030-75055-8_3

In this chapter, we offer an overview of methods and strategies via which genomics can influence everyday clinical practice with a particular focus on the impact these approaches can have on cardiovascular prevention.

Rare Variation Highlights Novel Disease Pathways

Background

Sequencing technologies have allowed for the discovery of rare coding variants that can lead to extreme deviations from normal phenotypes. The traditional approach to identify these variants starts with the finding of an extreme phenotype in the clinical setting. Once clinicians or researchers identify a person as an outlier for a specific condition, and assuming that phenomenon cannot be easily explained by an environmental factor or comorbidity, then they can perform what is formally known as a family linkage study [7]. Specifically, investigators can perform genotyping or sequencing of several affected and unaffected members of the family and evaluate how certain haplotypes segregate with presence of the target phenotype.

Relevance for Cardiovascular Prevention

This approach has been used successfully in cardiovascular prevention both clinically and in research. Perhaps the most widely appreciated recent example is the discovery of the PCSK9 gene as a major driver of atherosclerosis. In a series of studies, Boileaut et al. identified several families in France that had clear phenotypic signs of severe hypercholesterolemia with an autosomal dominant inheritance pattern but did not carry any mutations in LDLR or APOB, which at the time were the only known familial hypercholesterolemia (FH) genes. The investigators mapped the cause of these patients' hypercholesterolemia within chromosome 1 in a locus they named "FH3" [8]. They subsequently went further and with detailed experimental evidence they were able to identify with confidence that mutations in the PCSK9 gene were the cause of FH in these families [9]. This opened the door to a series of studies about PCSK9 inhibition as a potential new avenue for atherosclerotic cardiovascular disease (ASCVD) prevention that culminated to the creation of PCSK9 inhibitors evolocumab and alirocumab which are now widely used in clinical practice and have been proven to reduce both lipid levels and cardiovascular events [10, 11].

The discovery of other FH genes (APOE [12], ABCG5 [13], ABCG8 [13]) followed a similar path and we now are familiar with 8 genes that can cause FH and many more that can cause other subtypes of familial lipid disorders. Targeted gene sequencing is used in everyday practice to screen individuals at high risk for familial lipid disorders. The importance of diagnosing monogenic familial lipid disorders is twofold. First, it can guide therapy for the individual who is a mutation carrier. Specifically, we now know that people who have monogenic FH have a higher risk of disease than individuals with FH lacking any known mutation [14]. It is therefore prudent to treat LDL more aggressively in such patients. Second, it can inform evaluation and treatment of family members of the identified proband. Specifically, it is now recommended that we perform cascade screening in family members of individuals who have monogenic FH [15]. This approach can allow identification of asymptomatic individuals with FH who may benefit from early intervention to prevent ASCVD.

Beyond their influence in diagnosis and risk stratification, rare variants can help highlight novel disease pathways that can spark research into novel therapies for ASCVD as was the case for PCSK9. A more recent example of this approach is the identification of ANGPTL4. In a series of studies published in the *New England Journal of Medicine*, independent investigators identified rare coding variants of ANGPTL4, a gene that inhibits lipoprotein lipase, as risk factors for coronary artery disease [16, 17]. In the first of these studies, researchers evaluated the impact of rare coding variants across multiple genes in the genome in a high-throughput fashion in 72,000 cases with coronary disease and 120,000 controls. They discovered that inactivating variants of the ANGPTL4 gene confer protection against coronary disease potentially via lowering triglyceride levels [16]. An independent study published at around the same time confirmed these findings and also showed that the same ANGPTL4 variant leads to drastically lower triglyceride levels and higher HDL levels [17]. The researchers subsequently showed that monoclonal antibody inhibition of ANGPTL4 in mice and monkeys leads to decreased triglyceride levels [17], along with improved insulin sensitivity and glucose homeostasis [18]. In a similar design study, the same group of investigators showed that rare variants within ANGPTL3, a gene in the same family as ANGPTL4, also led to lower risk of coronary disease and decreased levels of all three lipid components (Triglycerides, LDL and HDL cholesterol). Monoclonal antibody inhibition of ANGPTL3 with a molecule named evinacumab decreased triglyceride levels by 76% and LDL cholesterol by 23% in humans [19]. Two subsequent phase 2 trials in individuals with homozygous FH [20] and refractory hypercholesterolemia [21] showed that evinacumab reduced LDL cholesterol by approximately 50% when added to standard of care therapy.

Beyond discovery of novel therapeutics, rare variant identification can also guide targeted therapy based on a mechanistic understanding of the defect that causes a certain disease phenotype. For example, we know that individuals with two copies of autosomal recessive ABCG8 or ABCG5 variants have a phenotype indistinguishable from FH [13]. These individuals have a condition known as sitosterolemia which leads to increased absorption and diminished bile secretion of plant sterols in the gut. This phenomenon in turn increases circulating levels of plant sterols that lead to increased LDL cholesterol measurements and premature coronary disease. Interestingly, plant sterol levels are not substantially affected by statin therapy, which is the first line treatment for most individuals with FH, but are instead particularly responsive to ezetimibe therapy. Ezetimibe decreases intestinal cholesterol absorption, making this medication a reasonable first line intervention for this group of patients [22].

Leveraging Common Variant Genomics to Understand Disease Pathophysiology

Background

It is increasingly understood that rare coding variants only account for a small portion of the heritability of most complex traits and diseases [23]. In contrast, a substantial portion of the heritability is driven by variants in non-coding regions of the genome [24]. Therefore, identification of these alternative disease-causing variants and their mechanism of action is a crucial task in our understanding of the genetic underpinnings of human disease. The genome-wide association (GWA) framework has been the workhorse method of investigations aiming to understand the way in which genetic variation influences disease risk. The last decade has seen a dramatic rise in the number of successful GWA studies (GWAS) performed. Indeed, the latest estimates from the GWAS catalog show that over 179,000 independent variant-trait associations have been identified by GWAS to-date [25].

The concept of GWAS is simple. Once we obtain the genotypes of a large set of individuals for whom we know the prevalence of a human disease, then we can associate each genotype individually with the risk of disease. The concept is similar to traditional cohort studies in which we associate an exposure with an outcome, only in this case the exposure is the genotype at a particular position in the DNA [26]. In contrast to traditional observational studies, this approach is more robust to reverse causation (as the genotype by definition precedes disease incidence) and some other confounding artifacts.

Although the GWAS strategy is simple in principle, it took several years for GWAS to become widespread [27]. The reasons behind this delay are variable. Firstly, there are often millions of genetic variants tested in each GWAS. Consequently, multiple testing burden is high and false positives are expected, which is why GWAS often require replication to have high confidence in detected associations. Further, although traditional confounding is uncommon in GWAS, these studies are prone to other sources of inference errors that are inherent to the way a GWAS is performed. Specifically, genotyping platforms and even more advanced whole genome sequencing technologies that are available nowadays can have errors [28]. These errors can happen in any stage across the genotyping process, from DNA isolation, to library preparation to the actual sequencing. Depending on the affected step, errors can either affect a single genotype from a single individual or can, not uncommonly, affect multiple participants and generate what is known as "batch effects" which if not corrected will inevitably lead to false GWAS results. Therefore, an extensive quality control procedure is necessary to successfully perform a GWAS. These quality control steps have now become standard practice [29]. GWAS studies are affected by another type of confounding known as population stratification [30]. Population stratification reflects the fact that different populations tend to have different ancestry and therefore substantial differences in their genotypes. The same populations also have different habits and are affected by different environmental factors. Therefore, these differences can confound the results of a GWAS. Approaches including Principal Component Analysis correction [31] and linear mixed models are now available to address these concerns. A detailed description of these is beyond the scope of the current review.

Last and perhaps most importantly, GWAS has been impeded by the fact that most common variants that are found in high enough numbers in a population to be able to be evaluated for association with disease, are also the same variants that are less likely to have large effects disease [32]. The reason for that becomes obvious when one considers evolutionary pressures. Variants that are likely to have major effects in disease are also likely to cause a fitness disadvantage and therefore be selected against. Consequently, for GWAS to successfully identify true genetic associations with disease, they require large numbers of enrolled individuals, as most common variants have only tiny effects on disease development.

Relevance for Cardiovascular Prevention

Despite these shortcomings, population genetics studies have been successful at identifying variants that play an important role in Cardiovascular Health. Indeed, there are presently over 160 identified loci across the genome that affect the risk of coronary artery disease [33] and a larger number of loci that influence lipid traits [34].

Beyond identification of these risk loci, functional characterization to dissect their mechanism of action is considered particularly important in the effort towards their clinical translation. In certain situations, the task is easy as the risk locus is found in a gene with a known function. For example, GWAS loci for coronary disease risk have been identified in the LDLR, PCSK9 and LPA genes. Even in these situations, GWAS can help expand our understanding of the impact of certain genes in disease. For example, a large multi-ethnic GWAS study in 2013 showed that variants near the LPA gene that affect lipoprotein (a) levels are strongly associated with aortic valve calcification and incident aortic stenosis, [35] thereby providing a novel target for the prevention of aortic valve stenosis.

However, in most cases the problem is more complicated because the GWAS locus is non-coding, and in some cases no nearby gene has a known role in disease development. A classic example is the discovery of SORT1. Early GWAS studies for coronary disease identified a locus in chromosome 1 that was inside an intron of the PSRC1 gene and that had a strong signal for association with disease, which replicated across multiple different cohorts. Initial studies attributed the effect of those variants to PSRC1 [36], a gene that is required for cell proliferation and normal progression through mitosis. However, a pivotal study from Musunuru et al. proved that to be a false assumption [37]. Despite the fact that the nearest gene for the variants identified in GWAS is indeed PSRC1, study of these variants in human hepatocytes showed that they do not in fact affect PSRC1 expression. Instead, the variants seemed to influence the expression of another more distant gene known as SORT1. The investigators subsequently performed experiments in mice in which they inactivated SORT1 using a small inhibitory RNA (siRNA) and showed that decreased SORT1 expression leads to an increase in the levels of LDL and VLDL by altering hepatic VLDL cholesterol secretion. SORT1 could therefore represent a potential novel drug target for ASCVD [38].

Many other examples exist in the literature of efforts to functionally characterize the role of identified ASCVD GWAS loci. In one case, investigators evaluated the role of a locus in chromosome 6 that is the second most significant GWAS association with coronary disease. They found that instead of the traditional hypothesis of the locus exerting its effects on ASCVD via an influence on the PHACTR1 gene, the locus actually has no impact on PHACTR1 but affects endothelin − 1 (EDN1), a more distant gene known to be associated with vascular stiffness [39]. In another example, researchers showed that a new gene known as LMOD1 is a major regulator of smooth muscle cell proliferation during the atherosclerotic process and fully explains the GWAS association with coronary disease in a chromosome 1 locus [40]. Lastly, a recent study by Lo Sardo et al. profiled and functionally characterized the most impactful coronary disease GWAS locus in 9p21 [41]. Using genome editing in inducible pluripotent stem cell (iPSC)-derived vascular smooth muscle cells (VSMCs), the investigators showed that VSMCs that carry the risk genotype demonstrate aberrant adhesion, contraction and proliferation, whereas activating the expression of a long non-coding RNA within the 9p21 locus known as ANRIL, induces risk phenotypes in non-risk VSMCs. This suggests that ANRIL may have a crucial role in increasing the risk of aberrant VSMC proliferation in atherosclerotic lesions.

Mendelian Randomization Can Help Us Understand Causal Relationships

Background

Beyond the role of genomics in propelling discovery of novel disease mechanisms, there are other important benefits that we can derive from genetic discoveries. A major advance of genomics in medical practice has been the application of Mendelian Randomization (MR) to understand causal factors in disease.

MR refers to the process by which we can leverage genotypes known to be directly linked to a specific exposure (for example genetic variants that affect LDL cholesterol levels) to randomize individuals into groups that subsequently allow us to test the effect of that exposure on outcomes of interest [42]. Indeed, the method is considered a tremendous advance to traditional observational cohort studies as it is much less prone to confounding and, provided certain basic assumptions hold, can allow us to infer causal relationships between exposures and outcomes before investing in an expensive and time-consuming randomized controlled trial [43].

Relevance for Cardiovascular Prevention

MR studies have been quite successful in identifying major underappreciated exposure-outcome relationships or disproving long-held beliefs in the field of Cardiovascular Prevention. For example, a large MR study performed in 2012 showed that genetic variants that lead to increased HDL cholesterol do not in fact confer protection against atherosclerosis [44], thereby providing a justification as to why previous randomized trials failed to show ASCVD prevention benefit from interventions that increase HDL cholesterol [45]. Similarly, different investigators performed MR to show that variants that directly affect inflammation via their influence on interleukin-6 (IL6) substantially increase the risk of adverse coronary events, thereby establishing the role of inflammation as a major risk factor for atherosclerosis [46]. This role was subsequently proven by a recent randomized trial that showed cardiovascular benefit from an intervention specifically targeting the innate immunity pathway for secondary prevention in patients with established ASCVD [47]. Similar to the above, MR studies have largely been successful at disentangling causal from non-causal factors for ASCVD. For example, multiple MR studies proved the role of increased blood pressure [48], increased LDL cholesterol [48, 49], triglycerides [50] and lipoprotein(a) [51] in coronary disease, whereas others failed to show a causal role of CETP [52] or vitamin D levels [53], effects largely confirmed by subsequent randomized trials.

Beyond associations that have already been tested and confirmed by randomized trials, MR studies can point towards a role for novel biomarkers and exposures in ASCVD risk, thereby providing new targets for therapeutic and preventive interventions. For example, a recent MR study demonstrated that ATP citrate lyase (ACLY), an enzyme that is found upstream of HMG-CoA reductase (HMGCR) in the cholesterol biosynthesis pathway is associated with a lipid effect and cardiovascular protection similar to HMGCR [54]. The lipid effect was shown in a randomized controlled trial of bempedoic acid, an inhibitor of ACLY, in which the active drug lowered LDL cholesterol when added to maximally tolerated statin therapy and did not lead to a higher incidence of adverse events [55].

Despite the indubitable success of MR studies in general, there are important caveats that demand cautious interpretation of their findings. Specifically, MR estimates are valid only if certain assumptions hold. Those assumptions are the following: (a) the genetic variants are associated with the exposure; (b) no unmeasured confounders are present in the association between the variants and the outcome; and (c) the variants affect the outcome only through their effect on the exposure. Even if all fundamental assumptions of MR hold, and MR does reveal a causal link between an exposure and an outcome, that cannot be construed as proof of what would happen in a randomized trial of an intervention aimed at targeting that same exposure. The reason for that is that interventions do not always have the same effect on the exposure as do the tested genetic variants. If their effects were exactly the same then an interpretation of MR as a mini-RCT is warranted but in the absence of that assertion, a more cautious interpretation would be that the MR findings represent unconfounded estimates of the impact of the exposure on the outcome [56]. One example that highlights this caveat of MR is found in recent trials of triglyceride-lowering regimens on ASCVD risk. MR studies from different groups have repeatedly shown that high triglycerides increase ASCVD risk [50, 57]. To capitalize on that, the recent STRENGTH randomized controlled trial [58] investigated the role of omega-3 fatty acids in ASCVD events. The study was terminated early for futility and showed that despite the significant decrease in triglyceride levels in omega-3 fatty acid recipients compared to corn-oil controls, ASCVD events were similar between the two groups. In contrast, the REDUCE-IT trial [59] which investigated isolated eicosapentaenoic acid (EPA) ethyl ester that also reduces triglycerides showed a significant reduction of ischemic events in the intervention group compared to placebo, hence highlighting how specific effects of different medications could lead to discordant findings despite promising MR studies.

Polygenic Risk Scores Can Improve Risk Prediction

Background

An important application of GWAS discoveries that has recently been appreciated is their role in predicting disease risk. Even in situations lacking a mechanistic understanding of the pathway that leads from GWAS variants to disease, we can still leverage the GWAS associations to generate polygenic risk scores for a disease [60]. These polygenic scores can subsequently be mapped to a probability of disease incidence and thus open the door to early identification of individuals at risk for a particular disease by genotyping or sequencing their genome, which could prove highly beneficial in instituting early prevention or treatment.

There are several considerations that should be taken into account when creating a polygenic risk score for a particular disease. One of the major challenges lies in the fact that nearby variants tend to be highly correlated with each other (a phenomenon known as linkage disequilibrium or LD that arises due to historical patterns of recombination events in the human population). Consequently, for any given disease risk variant identified in a GWAS, often hundreds or thousands of nearby variants will also appear to be significantly associated with the disease in the same GWAS, although none of these associated variants actually have any causal phenotypic consequences [61]. Therefore, there have been substantial research efforts on developing methodologies that can generate a robust polygenic risk score without overcounting associations that happen to occur within genomic regions of high LD. The traditional approach has been what is known as pruning and thresholding [62]. In this approach, we incorporate into the polygenic risk scores only associations that pass the genome-wide significant p-value threshold of $5*10^{-8}$ and among correlated variants (in LD) we select one variant (traditionally the variant with the strongest GWA signal) to enter into the polygenic score. Although this approach has been successful at predicting disease risk, more recent approaches that leverage sub-threshold loci and/or use a larger number of variants weighted by a metric associated with their pairwise LD have been able to achieve higher predictive power [63, 64].

Another important issue related to the above has to do with the fact that LD patterns are usually different among different ethnic groups. Consequently, polygenic risk scores generated based on European GWAS, which are by far the most prevalent and highly powered, lose in predictive capacity when applied to non-European ethnic groups [65]. Although adjustments of the polygenic risk scores to account for ethnicity have been proposed [66], all existing approaches have limitations and, in the absence of large scale highly powered GWAS for all different ethnic populations, a widely applicable solution to that problem remains elusive.

Relevance for Cardiovascular Prevention

Calculating the risk of ASCVD for a given individual has been in the spotlight of preventive cardiology for several years. Indeed multiple studies have tried to combine different demographic characteristics, comorbid conditions and biomarkers to predict the individual risk of disease and this type of risk estimation is used in everyday practice to guide primary prevention interventions, such as lipid lowering therapies in the form of the AHA Pooled Cohort Equation [67] or the European SCORE system [68].

Polygenic risk scores offer a novel attractive method of calculating risk of ASCVD that could have substantial implications for clinical practice. Although the cardiovascular medicine community has identified family history as a risk factor for ASCVD for several years, only recently did investigators appreciate the fact that family history is a poor surrogate for polygenic risk prediction [69], which led to an increased interest in other approaches to calculate inherited risk [70]. Initial efforts at using results from large scale GWAS studies for coronary disease in calculating inherited risk for ASCVD took the approach of selecting only genome-wide significant variants (those with p-value $< 5*10^{-8}$) for inclusion in the risk estimation [71]. Although these efforts were successful, newer approaches that leverage signal across the entire genome by incorporating a much larger number of variants [72] or even all tested GWAS variants [73], weighted in a way that accounts for the underlying LD structure, are much more effective in robustly estimating the downstream risk of disease. Indeed, research groups have now shown that polygenic risk scores for ASCVD can predict risk of disease beyond and additively to lifestyle factors [74], whereas recent post-hoc analyses of the FOURIER [75] and ODYSSEY OUTCOMES [76] trials showed that a high polygenic risk for coronary disease can predict individuals who have a higher benefit from PCSK9 inhibitor treatment, regardless of their clinical risk factors. More importantly, a polygenic risk score is acquired at birth and can therefore provide a reliable estimator of ASCVD risk well in advance of any other prediction systems that rely on biomarkers or comorbid conditions, and very strongly on age.

There remain, however, several questions about polygenic risk score use that could determine the scope and strategy of implementation into clinical practice. First, in their current form, polygenic risk scores for ASCVD are heavily affected by ancestry. Since most GWAS studies that guide polygenic risk score generation have been performed on European participants, it is not a surprise that polygenic risk scores for most diseases, including ASCVD are more reliable in European ancestry individuals. That is not to say that the application of an ASCVD polygenic score generated from a European GWAS is useless in individuals of other race groups, but their predictive power is somewhat reduced [77]. Second, most current versions of polygenic risk scores include only common variants. Consequently, additional components that substantially change the heritable risk of ASCVD, such as PCSK9, APOB or LDLR rare variants, are not presently incorporated in these risk scores. Last but not least, it remains uncertain what clinical benefit can be derived in practice from the knowledge of a high or low polygenic score for ASCVD. Although the literature has shown that a high polygenic risk score (top 5th percentile) for coronary disease confers similar risk of downstream events to a clinical diagnosis of familial hypercholesterolemia [77], and retrospective studies support the notion that individuals in those extremes of polygenic risk have greater benefit from lipid lowering agents, randomized data confirming that benefit are still lacking. In fact, recent studies in independent large population genetics cohorts show that even robustly estimated polygenic scores for coronary disease do not outperform traditional risk stratification measures like the Pooled Cohort Equation in middle aged European ancestry individuals and have a minimal, if any, additive prediction benefit with questionable clinical significance [78, 79]. Further, although the biggest strength of polygenic risk score may be its ability to predict risk of disease at a young age [70], data on timing of intervention for patients in extremes of polygenic risk are absent to date. With the growing use and availability of sequencing technologies, along with the decreasing associated cost (current genotyping cost per person is < $100) it is likely that many of these questions will be answered in the near future.

Conclusions and Future Perspectives

There is no doubt that the era of genomic revolution will influence Cardiovascular Prevention in a major way. Many of its effects are already seen in multiple aspects of everyday practice, including the discovery of novel disease pathways and treatment targets, the improved understanding of causal relationships via MR and the strengthened risk stratification via the discovery of genetic variants that affect risk of disease (Table 1). As more aspects of the effects of our genetic code on cardiovascular disease become known and as broader sequencing availability will allow for incorporation of genetic predictions in clinical trials, it is likely that we will be seeing an increasing clinical use of these discoveries in the near future. Private companies are already making genetic tools commercially available and it is paramount for the medical community to provide guidelines for their appropriate use and interpretation. In summary, the recent computational biology advances, along with the discovery of methods to edit human DNA at a nucleotide resolution may harbor an era where genomic medicine can grow from a peripheral tool in the disposal of clinicians and researchers to the predominant driver of precision medical diagnosis, prevention and treatment.

Table 1 Genomic methods that affect cardiovascular disease prevention

Method	Advantages	Limitations	Examples of application to Preventive Cardiology
Family linkage studies	Allow for rare variant identification—can discover new disease-risk genes	Low throughput, explain only a small portion of disease heritability	PCSK9 gene discovery
Genome-wide association studies	High-throughput discoveries of variants associated with risk of disease	Interpretation is hard and require substantial downstream functional characterization. Difficult to use for rare variants	Discovery of SORT1
Mendelian randomization studies	Allow for the study of causal relationships between exposures and disease. Are not affected by reverse causation	Require certain assumptions to hold	Discovery of ACLY
Polygenic risk scores	Allow for disease risk stratification—often additive to traditional disease risk factors	Limited generalizability to multi-ethnic populations, cost of sequencing	Polygenic score for CAD has equivalent risk of disease to a diagnosis of familial hypercholesterolemia

ACLY: ATP-citrate lyase, CAD: Coronary artery disease, PCSK9: Paraprotein convertase subtilisin/kexin type 9, SORT1: Sortilin-1

References

1. Hunkapiller T, Kaiser RJ, Koop BF, et al. Large-scale and automated DNA sequence determination. Science. 1991;254(5028):59–67. https://doi.org/10.1126/science.1925562.
2. Koboldt DC, Steinberg KM, Larson DE, et al. The next-generation sequencing revolution and its impact on genomics. Cell. 2013;155(1):27–38. https://doi.org/10.1016/j.cell.2013.09.006.
3. Smith DR. Goodbye genome paper, hello genome report: the increasing popularity of 'genome announcements' and their impact on science. Brief Funct Genomics. 2017;16 (3):156–62. https://doi.org/10.1093/bfgp/elw026.
4. Zhang H, Klareskog L, Matussek A, et al. Translating genomic medicine to the clinic: challenges and opportunities. Genome Med. 2019;11(1):9–1. https://doi.org/10.1186/s13073-019-0622-1.
5. Anonymous. A randomized, controlled trial of aspirin in persons recovered from myocardial infarction. JAMA. 1980;243(7):661–9.
6. Evidence-Based Medicine Working Group. Evidence-based medicine. A new approach to teaching the practice of medicine. JAMA 1992;268(17):2420–5. https://doi.org/10.1001/jama.1992.03490170092032.
7. Borecki IB, Province MA. Genetic and genomic discovery using family studies. Circulation. 2008;118(10):1057–63. https://doi.org/10.1161/CIRCULATIONAHA.107.714592.
8. Varret M, Rabes JP, Saint-Jore B et al. A third major locus for autosomal dominant hypercholesterolemia maps to 1p34.1-p32. Am J Hum Genet. 64(5):1378–87. S0002–9297 (07)62283–6 [pii].
9. Abifadel M, Varret M, Rabes JP, et al. Mutations in PCSK9 cause autosomal dominant hypercholesterolemia. Nat Genet. 2003;34(2):154–6. https://doi.org/10.1038/ng1161.
10. Sabatine MS, Giugliano RP, Keech AC, et al. Evolocumab and clinical outcomes in patients with cardiovascular disease. N Engl J Med. 2017;376(18):1713–22. https://doi.org/10.1056/NEJMoa1615664.
11. Schwartz GG, Steg PG, Szarek M, et al. Alirocumab and Cardiovascular outcomes after acute coronary syndrome. N Engl J Med. 2018;379(22):2097–107. https://doi.org/10.1056/NEJMoa1801174.
12. Awan Z, Choi HY, Stitziel N et al. APOE p.Leu167del mutation in familial hypercholesterolemia. Atherosclerosis 231(2):218–22. https://doi.org/10.1016/j.atherosclerosis.2013.09.007.
13. Berge KE, Tian H, Graf GA et al. Accumulation of dietary cholesterol in sitosterolemia caused by mutations in adjacent ABC transporters. Science 2000;290(5497):1771–1775. 9022 [pii].
14. Trinder M, Li X, DeCastro ML et al. Risk of premature atherosclerotic disease in patients with monogenic versus polygenic familial hypercholesterolemia. J Am Coll Cardiol. 2019;74 (4):512–22. S0735–1097(19)35378–1 [pii].
15. Sturm AC, Knowles JW, Gidding SS et al. Clinical genetic testing for familial hypercholesterolemia: JACC scientific expert panel. J Am Coll Cardiol. 2018;72(6):662–80. S0735–1097 (18)35065–4 [pii].
16. Myocardial Infarction Genetics and CARDIoGRAM Exome Consortia Investigators, Stitziel NO, Stirrups KE et al. Coding Variation in ANGPTL4, LPL, and SVEP1 and the Risk of Coronary Disease. N Engl J Med. 2016;374(12):1134–1144. https://doi.org/10.1056/NEJMoa1507652.
17. Dewey FE, Gusarova V, O'Dushlaine C, et al. Inactivating variants in ANGPTL4 and risk of coronary artery disease. N Engl J Med. 2016;374(12):1123–33. https://doi.org/10.1056/NEJMoa1510926.
18. Gusarova V, O'Dushlaine C, Teslovich TM et al. Genetic inactivation of ANGPTL4 improves glucose homeostasis and is associated with reduced risk of diabetes. Nat Commun. 2018;9 (1):2252-z. https://doi.org/10.1038/s41467-018-04611-z.

19. Dewey FE, Gusarova V, Dunbar RL, et al. Genetic and pharmacologic inactivation of ANGPTL3 and cardiovascular disease. N Engl J Med. 2017;377(3):211–21. https://doi.org/10.1056/NEJMoa1612790.

20. Raal FJ, Rosenson RS, Reeskamp LF, et al. Evinacumab for homozygous familial hypercholesterolemia. N Engl J Med. 2020;383(8):711–20. https://doi.org/10.1056/NEJMoa2004215.

21. Rosenson RS, Burgess LJ, Ebenbichler CF, et al. Evinacumab in patients with refractory hypercholesterolemia. N Engl J Med. 2020;383(24):2307–19. https://doi.org/10.1056/NEJMoa2031049.

22. Salen G, von Bergmann K, Lutjohann D, et al. Ezetimibe effectively reduces plasma plant sterols in patients with sitosterolemia. Circulation. 2004;109(8):966–71. https://doi.org/10.1161/01.CIR.0000116766.31036.03.

23. International Multiple Sclerosis Genetics Consortium Electronic address: chris cotsapas@yale edu, International Multiple Sclerosis Genetics Consortium (2018) Low-Frequency and Rare-Coding Variation Contributes to Multiple Sclerosis Risk. Cell 2018;175(6):1679–87.e7. S0092–8674(18)31261–3 [pii].

24. Zhang F, Lupski JR. Non-coding genetic variants in human disease. Hum Mol Genet. 2015;24 (R1):102. https://doi.org/10.1093/hmg/ddv259.

25. Buniello A, MacArthur JAL, Cerezo M, et al. The NHGRI-EBI GWAS catalog of published genome-wide association studies, targeted arrays and summary statistics 2019. Nucleic Acids Res. 2019;47(D1):D1005–12. https://doi.org/10.1093/nar/gky1120.

26. Tam V, Patel N, Turcotte M, et al. Benefits and limitations of genome-wide association studies. Nat Rev Genet. 2019;20(8):467–84. https://doi.org/10.1038/s41576-019-0127-1.

27. McClellan J, King MC. Genetic heterogeneity in human disease. Cell. 2010;141(2):210–7. https://doi.org/10.1016/j.cell.2010.03.032.

28. Pompanon F, Bonin A, Bellemain E et al. Genotyping errors: causes, consequences and solutions. Nat Rev Genet. 2005;6(11):847–59. nrg1707 [pii].

29. Turner S, Armstrong LL, Bradford Y et al. Quality control procedures for genome-wide association studies. Curr Protoc Hum Genet. 2011; Chapter 1:Unit 1.19. https://doi.org/10.1002/0471142905.hg0119s68.

30. Hellwege JN, Keaton JM, Giri A et al. Population Stratification in genetic association studies. Curr Protoc Hum Genet. 2017;95:1.22.1–1.22.23. https://doi.org/10.1002/cphg.48

31. Price AL, Patterson NJ, Plenge RM et al. Principal components analysis corrects for stratification in genome-wide association studies. Nat Genet. 2006;38(8):904–909. ng1847 [pii].

32. Park JH, Gail MH, Weinberg CR, et al. Distribution of allele frequencies and effect sizes and their interrelationships for common genetic susceptibility variants. Proc Natl Acad Sci USA. 2011;108(44):18026–31. https://doi.org/10.1073/pnas.1114759108.

33. van der Harst P, Verweij N. Identification of 64 novel genetic Loci provides an expanded view on the genetic architecture of coronary artery disease. Circ Res. 2018;122(3):433–43. https://doi.org/10.1161/CIRCRESAHA.117.312086.

34. Hoffmann TJ, Theusch E, Haldar T, et al. A large electronic-health-record-based genome-wide study of serum lipids. Nat Genet. 2018;50(3):401–13. https://doi.org/10.1038/s41588-018-0064-5.

35. Thanassoulis G, Campbell CY, Owens DS, et al. Genetic associations with valvular calcification and aortic stenosis. N Engl J Med. 2013;368(6):503–12. https://doi.org/10.1056/NEJMoa1109034.

36. Samani NJ, Erdmann J, Hall AS et al. Genomewide association analysis of coronary artery disease. N Engl J Med. 2007;357(5):443–53. NEJMoa072366 [pii].

37. Musunuru K, Strong A, Frank-Kamenetsky M, et al. From noncoding variant to phenotype via SORT1 at the 1p13 cholesterol locus. Nature. 2010;466(7307):714–9. https://doi.org/10.1038/nature09266.

38. Goettsch C, Kjolby M, Aikawa E. Sortilin and its multiple roles in cardiovascular and metabolic diseases. Arterioscler Thromb Vasc Biol. 2018;38(1):19–25. https://doi.org/10.1161/ATVBAHA.117.310292.

39. Gupta RM, Hadaya J, Trehan A et al. A genetic variant associated with five vascular diseases is a distal regulator of endothelin-1 gene expression. Cell 2017;170(3):522–33.e15. S0092-8674(17)30768-7 [pii].

40. Nanda V, Wang T, Pjanic M, et al. Functional regulatory mechanism of smooth muscle cell-restricted LMOD1 coronary artery disease locus. PLoS Genet. 2018;14(11). https://doi.org/10.1371/journal.pgen.1007755.

41. Lo Sardo V, Chubukov P, Ferguson W et al. Unveiling the role of the most impactful cardiovascular risk locus through haplotype editing. Cell 2018;175(7):1796–810.e20. S0092-8674(18)31506-X [pii].

42. Emdin CA, Khera AV, Kathiresan S. Mendelian randomization. JAMA. 2017;318(19):1925–6. https://doi.org/10.1001/jama.2017.17219.

43. Sheehan NA, Didelez V, Burton PR, et al. Mendelian randomisation and causal inference in observational epidemiology. PLoS Med. 2008;5(8). https://doi.org/10.1371/journal.pmed.0050177.

44. Voight BF, Peloso GM, Orho-Melander M, et al. Plasma HDL cholesterol and risk of myocardial infarction: a mendelian randomisation study. Lancet. 2012;380(9841):572–80. https://doi.org/10.1016/S0140-6736(12)60312-2.

45. Investigators AIM-HIGH, Boden WE, Probstfield JL, et al. Niacin in patients with low HDL cholesterol levels receiving intensive statin therapy. N Engl J Med. 2011;365(24):2255–67. https://doi.org/10.1056/NEJMoa1107579.

46. Interleukin-6 Receptor Mendelian Randomisation Analysis (IL6R MR) Consortium, Swerdlow DI, Holmes MV et al (2012) The interleukin-6 receptor as a target for prevention of coronary heart disease: a mendelian randomisation analysis. Lancet 2012;379(9822):1214–1224. https://doi.org/10.1016/S0140-6736(12)60110-X [doi]

47. Ridker PM, Everett BM, Thuren T, et al. Antiinflammatory therapy with canakinumab for atherosclerotic disease. N Engl J Med. 2017;377(12):1119–31. https://doi.org/10.1056/NEJMoa1707914.

48. Ference BA, Bhatt DL, Catapano AL, et al. Association of genetic variants related to combined exposure to lower low-density lipoproteins and lower systolic blood pressure with lifetime risk of cardiovascular disease. JAMA. 2019. https://doi.org/10.1001/jama.2019.14120.

49. Waterworth DM, Ricketts SL, Song K, et al. Genetic variants influencing circulating lipid levels and risk of coronary artery disease. Arterioscler Thromb Vasc Biol. 2010;30(11):2264–76. https://doi.org/10.1161/ATVBAHA.109.201020.

50. Holmes MV, Asselbergs FW, Palmer TM, et al. Mendelian randomization of blood lipids for coronary heart disease. Eur Heart J. 2015;36(9):539–50. https://doi.org/10.1093/eurheartj/eht571.

51. Burgess S, Ference BA, Staley JR, et al. Association of LPA Variants with risk of coronary disease and the implications for lipoprotein(a)-lowering therapies: a mendelian randomization analysis. JAMA Cardiol. 2018;3(7):619–27. https://doi.org/10.1001/jamacardio.2018.1470.

52. Millwood IY, Bennett DA, Holmes MV, et al. Association of CETP gene variants with risk for vascular and nonvascular diseases among chinese adults. JAMA Cardiol. 2018;3(1):34–43. https://doi.org/10.1001/jamacardio.2017.4177.

53. Manousaki D, Mokry LE, Ross S, et al. Mendelian randomization studies do not support a role for vitamin D in coronary artery disease. Circ Cardiovasc Genet. 2016;9(4):349–56. https://doi.org/10.1161/CIRCGENETICS.116.001396[doi].

54. Ference BA, Ray KK, Catapano AL, et al. Mendelian randomization study of ACLY and cardiovascular disease. N Engl J Med. 2019;380(11):1033–42. https://doi.org/10.1056/NEJMoa1806747.

55. Ray KK, Bays HE, Catapano AL, et al. Safety and efficacy of bempedoic acid to reduce ldl cholesterol. N Engl J Med. 2019;380(11):1022–32. https://doi.org/10.1056/NEJMoa1803917.

56. Sun YQ, Burgess S, Staley JR, et al. Body mass index and all cause mortality in HUNT and UK Biobank studies: linear and non-linear mendelian randomisation analyses. BMJ. 2019;364. https://doi.org/10.1136/bmj.l1042.
57. Allara E, Morani G, Carter P, et al. genetic determinants of lipids and cardiovascular disease outcomes: a wide-angled mendelian randomization investigation. Circ Genom Precis Med. 2019;12(12). https://doi.org/10.1161/CIRCGEN.119.002711.
58. Nicholls SJ, Lincoff AM, Garcia M, et al. Effect of high-dose Omega-3 Fatty acids vs corn oil on major adverse cardiovascular events in patients at high cardiovascular risk: the STRENGTH randomized clinical trial. JAMA. 2020;324(22):2268–80. https://doi.org/10.1001/jama.2020.22258.
59. Bhatt DL, Steg PG, Miller M, et al. Cardiovascular risk reduction with Icosapent ethyl for Hypertriglyceridemia. N Engl J Med. 2019;380(1):11–22. https://doi.org/10.1056/NEJMoa1812792.
60. Richardson TG, Harrison S, Hemani G, et al. An atlas of polygenic risk score associations to highlight putative causal relationships across the human phenome. Elife. 2019;8. https://doi.org/10.7554/eLife.43657.10.7554/eLife.43657.
61. Ardlie KG, Kruglyak L, Seielstad M. Patterns of linkage disequilibrium in the human genome. Nat Rev Genet. 2002;3(4):299–309. https://doi.org/10.1038/nrg777.
62. Choi SW, Heng Mak TS, O'Reilly PF. A guide to performing Polygenic Risk Score analyses; 2018. bioRxiv:416545. https://doi.org/10.1101/416545
63. Vilhjalmsson BJ, Yang J, Finucane HK, et al. Modeling linkage disequilibrium increases accuracy of polygenic risk scores. Am J Hum Genet. 2015;97(4):576–92. https://doi.org/10.1016/j.ajhg.2015.09.001.
64. Prive F, Vilhjalmsson BJ, Aschard H et al. Making the most of clumping and thresholding for polygenic scores. Am J Hum Genet. 2019;105(6):1213–21. S0002-9297(19)30422-7 [pii].
65. Duncan L, Shen H, Gelaye B, et al. Analysis of polygenic risk score usage and performance in diverse human populations. Nat Commun. 2019;10(1):3328. https://doi.org/10.1038/s41467-019-11112-0.
66. Marquez-Luna C, Loh PR, South Asian Type 2 Diabetes (SAT2D) Consortium et al. Multiethnic polygenic risk scores improve risk prediction in diverse populations. Genet Epidemiol. 2017;41(8):811–23. https://doi.org/10.1002/gepi.22083
67. Ridker PM, Cook NR (2016) The pooled cohort equations 3 years on: building a stronger foundation. Circulation 2016;134(23):1789–91. CIRCULATIONAHA.116.024246 [pii].
68. Conroy RM, Pyorala K, Fitzgerald AP et al. Estimation of ten-year risk of fatal cardiovascular disease in Europe: the SCORE project. Eur Heart J. 2003;24(11):987–1003. S0195668X03001143 [pii].
69. Tada H, Melander O, Louie JZ, et al. Risk prediction by genetic risk scores for coronary heart disease is independent of self-reported family history. Eur Heart J. 2016;37(6):561–7. https://doi.org/10.1093/eurheartj/ehv462.
70. Natarajan P. Polygenic risk scoring for coronary heart disease: the first risk factor. J Am Coll Cardiol. 2018;72(16):1894–7. S0735-1097(18)36946-8 [pii].
71. Mega JL, Stitziel NO, Smith JG, et al. Genetic risk, coronary heart disease events, and the clinical benefit of statin therapy: an analysis of primary and secondary prevention trials. Lancet. 2015;385(9984):2264–71. https://doi.org/10.1016/S0140-6736(14)61730-X.
72. Inouye M, Abraham G, Nelson CP et al. Genomic risk prediction of coronary artery disease in 480,000 adults: implications for primary prevention. J Am Coll Cardiol. 2018;72(16):1883–93. S0735-1097(18)36949-3 [pii].
73. Khera AV, Chaffin M, Aragam KG, et al. Genome-wide polygenic scores for common diseases identify individuals with risk equivalent to monogenic mutations. Nat Genet. 2018;50(9):1219–24. https://doi.org/10.1038/s41588-018-0183-z.
74. Khera AV, Emdin CA, Drake I, et al. Genetic risk, adherence to a healthy lifestyle, and coronary disease. N Engl J Med. 2016;375(24):2349–58. https://doi.org/10.1056/NEJMoa1605086.

75. Marston NA, Kamanu FK, Nordio F, et al. Predicting benefit from evolocumab therapy in patients with atherosclerotic disease using a genetic risk score: results from the FOURIER trial. Circulation. 2020;141(8):616–23. https://doi.org/10.1161/CIRCULATIONAHA.119.043805.

76. Damask A, Steg PG, Schwartz GG, et al. Patients with high genome-wide polygenic risk scores for coronary artery disease may receive greater clinical benefit from Alirocumab treatment in the ODYSSEY OUTCOMES trial. Circulation. 2020;141(8):624–36. https://doi.org/10.1161/CIRCULATIONAHA.119.044434.

77. Khera AV, Chaffin M, Zekavat SM, et al. Whole-genome sequencing to characterize monogenic and polygenic contributions in patients hospitalized with early-onset myocardial infarction. Circulation. 2019;139(13):1593–602. https://doi.org/10.1161/CIRCULATIONAHA.118.035658.

78. Mosley JD, Gupta DK, Tan J, et al. Predictive accuracy of a polygenic risk score compared with a clinical risk score for incident coronary heart disease. JAMA. 2020;323(7):627–35. https://doi.org/10.1001/jama.2019.21782.

79. Elliott J, Bodinier B, Bond TA, et al. Predictive accuracy of a polygenic risk score-enhanced Prediction model vs a clinical risk score for coronary artery disease. JAMA. 2020;323(7):636–45. https://doi.org/10.1001/jama.2019.22241[doi].

Atherosclerosis Imaging

Omar Dzaye, Cara Reiter-Brennan, and Michael J. Blaha

Abbreviations

ABI	Ankle-brachial index
ACC/AHA	American College of Cardiology/American Heart Association
ACS	Acute coronary syndrome
ASCVD	Atherosclerotic cardiovascular disease
AUC	Area under the curve
CAC	Coronary artery calcium
CAD	Coronary artery disease
CCTA	Coronary computed tomography angiography
CHD	Coronary heart disease
CI	Confidence interval
CIMT	Carotid intima media thickness
CMR	Cardiac magnetic resonance
CONFIRM	COroNary CT Angiography Evaluation For Clinical Outcomes: An InteRnational Multicenter Registry
CRESCENT	Computed Tomography vs. Exercise Testing in Suspected Coronary Artery Disease
CT	Computed tomography
CVD	Cardiovascular disease
DHS	Dallas Heart Study
DIAD	Detection of Ischemia in Asymptomatic Diabetics
EBCT	Elector-beam computed tomography
ECC	Extra-coronary calcification
ESC	European Society of Cardiology
HNR	Heinz Nixdorf Recall

O. Dzaye · C. Reiter-Brennan · M. J. Blaha (✉)
Johns Hopkins Ciccarone Center for Prevention of Cardiovascular Disease, Johns Hopkins University School of Medicine, Baltimore, MD, US
e-mail: mblaha1@jhmi.edu

O. Dzaye
Russell H. Morgan Department of Radiology and Radiological Science, Johns Hopkins University School of Medicine, Baltimore, MD, US

© Springer Nature Switzerland AG 2021
S. S. Martin (ed.), *Precision Medicine in Cardiovascular Disease Prevention*,
https://doi.org/10.1007/978-3-030-75055-8_4

HR	Hazard ratio
hsCRP	High sensitivity C-reactive protein
LDL-C	Low-density lipoprotein cholesterol
LV	Left ventricular
MACE	Major adverse cardiovascular events
MDCT	Multidetector computed tomographic scanners
MESA	Multi Ethnic-Study of Atherosclerosis
MI	Myocardial infarction
MPI	Myocardial perfusion imaging
MRI	Magnetic resonance imaging
NNH	Number needed to harm
NNT	Number needed to treat
NRI	Net reclassification improvement
NT-proBNP	N-terminal-pro hormone B-type natriuretic peptide
PCE	Pooled cohort equations
PET	Positron emission tomography
PROMISE	Prospective Multicenter Imaging Study for Evaluation of Chest Pain
SCOT-HEART	Scottish Computed Tomography of the Heart
SPECT	Single photon emission computed tomography
USPSTF	United States Preventive Services Task Force

Traditional Risk Scores and Individualized Risk Assessment

Traditional cardiovascular risk assessment is defined by the routine screening of individuals without symptoms of cardiovascular disease (CVD) for risk factors in order to detect increased CVD risk [1]. Detection of risk rather than exclusion of clinical CVD is emphasized. This traditional approach to screening is widely endorsed by general practice guidelines, including the United States Preventive Services Task Force (USPSTF) guidelines. These guidelines recommend routine screening of middle aged adults using only widely available traditional atherosclerotic cardiovascular disease (ASCVD) risk factors, such as blood cholesterol levels and blood pressure [2]. Multiple risk models have been developed for quantifying traditional cardiovascular risk assessment. Perhaps most widely known in the United States, the 2013 American College of Cardiology/American Heart Association (ACC/AHA) guidelines published the Pooled Cohort Equations (PCE) which model the 10-year risk of a first ASCVD event (heart attack, stroke, or cardiovascular death) [3]. Accordingly, current 2018 ACC/AHA cholesterol management guidelines and 2019 ACC/AHA primary prevention guidelines carried PCE forward [4, 5]. Similar to most other cardiovascular risk assessment scores, the PCE calculates risk by taking into account traditional risk factors, such as smoking status, sex, race, systolic blood pressure, cholesterol, diabetes, and age.

Most cardiovascular risk calculators have been developed to guide preventive therapy decisions for individuals. However, risk calculators estimate the average risk of a population with similar risk factors, and thus might better estimate the net benefit of preventive therapy across a broad population [1]. Thus, the risk estimate and consequent clinical decision making for the individual—not the population at large—may be less accurate using these population-based models [1]. Therefore, ACC/AHA guidelines as well as the European Society of Cardiology (ESC) guidelines also have provisions for arriving at a more individualized approach to risk assessment. Individualized risk assessment aims to optimize risk assessment of the individual patient rather than rely exclusively on the broad population average estimate (Fig. 1). With this approach, a patient's risk status can be re-classified from the traditional risk factor-only models. This is particularly useful in individuals with intermediate cardiovascular risk by traditional risk models, where risk-based clinical decision making may be uncertain.

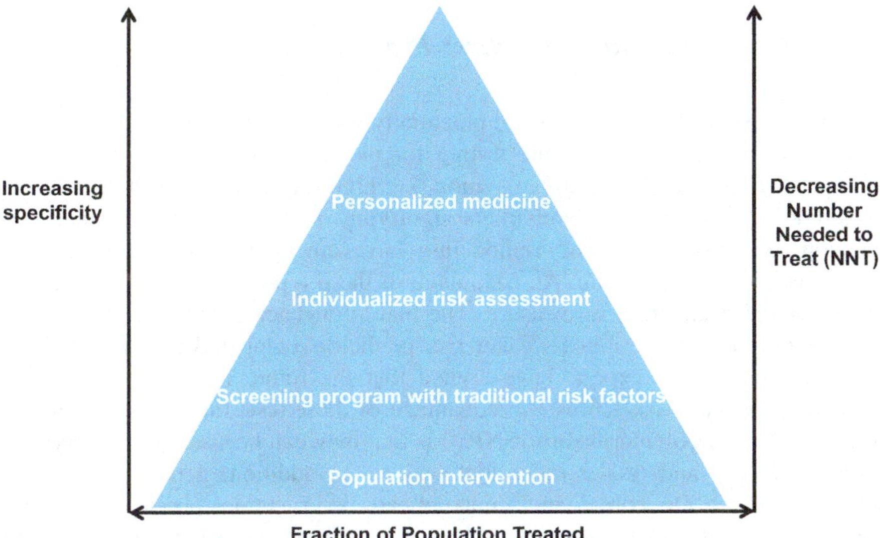

Fig. 1 Adapted from Michos et al. Screening for Atherosclerotic Cardiovascular Disease in Asymptomatic Individuals, 2018, Chronic Coronary Artery Disease: A Companion to Braunwald's Heart Disease (pp. 459–478). Population-based versus individual based approaches to preventive therapy: selection of target groups. The number needed to treat (NNT) decreases and specificity increases as the treatment spectrum narrows from population-based to individual-based approaches. NNT = number needed to treat

For example, patients in whom a more individualized approach results in de-risking (lowering the post-test risk estimate after applying the individualized approach) might safely avoid pharmacological primary prevention, even though they would have qualified for aggressive treatment based on traditional risk assessment with conventional risk factors. In contrast, sometimes an individualized approach might identify unheralded risk that could not be arrived at by conventional risk factors alone, necessitating aggressive preventive pharmacologic intervention.

While many strategies for individualized risk assessment exist, this chapter will focus on imaging of subclinical atherosclerosis to help refine personalization of risk estimates. This is because imaging allows direct detection of the precursor lesion (atherosclerotic plaque) in an individual in the arterial bed of interest. Imaging produces results more akin to a "disease score" rather than a traditional risk factor. While multiple imaging modalities exist, computed tomography (CT) imaging appears to be a highly effective tool in order to quantify atherosclerotic burden, and is most ready for routine clinical practice. Detection of coronary artery calcium (CAC) through a non-contrast cardiac-gated CT or the visualization of the coronary arteries through contrasted CT angiography (CTA) can effectively quantify cardiovascular risk.

Proposed Tools for Personalizing Risk Estimation

Serum Biomarkers and Genetics: Pros and Cons

The optimal strategy to test the large potentially at-risk population is controversial. Many have advocated for routine testing for blood-based serum biomarkers, for example tests for subclinical inflammation (i.e. high sensitivity C-reactive protein). In addition, multiple other biomarkers signifying oxidative stress, vascular dysfunction, or myocardial injury/remodeling have emerged as supplying varying incremental prognostic value. An advantage of these types of tests is that they are relatively cheap and easy to measure. The main drawback is that they lack specificity, and generally are much weaker risk predictors compared to atherosclerosis imaging. Many other experts have argued that the future is genetics, including so-called polygenic risk scores. An advantage of these tests (at least as individual single nucleotide polymorphisms (SNPs)) is that they can be specific to underlying pathophysiology and to the individual patient. In addition, genetics allow risk detection early in life, consequently making early interventions possible. However, the downside is that they are costly, not widely available, not strong risk predictors as individual SNPs, and that they lose their specificity for underlying pathophysiology when combined into polygenic risk scores.

Here we consider the example of serum measurements of natriuretic peptides. Evidence suggests that natriuretic peptide levels may be increased in pre-clinical heart failure, and therefore may predict future heart failure or cardiovascular death.

For instance, participants reclassified to Stage B heart failure from Stage A heart failure had significantly higher N-terminal-pro hormone B-type natriuretic peptide (NT-proBNP) than other stage B HF patients [6]. However, the optimal threshold marking elevated risk for NT-proBNP is not yet established [7]. A matter of consideration is also the lower levels of NT-proBNP in obese patients, reducing the diagnostic sensitivity in these populations [7]. NT-proBNP is also highly linked to age, with increasing value found throughout adult life, once again making interpretation more challenging. Clinical trials have not been able to show that NT-proBNP-guided management reduces the risk of initial or recurrent heart failure [8, 9].

Combining multiple biomarkers may still be a viable approach to guiding preventive therapy in the future [10]. However, biomarker panels have so far led to relatively disappointing results in terms of risk discrimination [11, 12]. Several studies have also evaluated combination of imaging with biomarkers to enhance diagnostic testing [13, 14]. For instance, the combination of NT-proBNP with echocardiography was shown to effectively reclassify 5-year heart failure risk of older adults when added to clinical models [14].

Coronary Artery Calcium

CAC Imaging

Early imaging modalities relied on chest radiography as well as fluoroscopy or digital subtraction fluoroscopy to see CAC [15]. Later, more precise quantification of CAC became possible with the introduction of cardiac gating for electron-beam computed tomography (EBCT) [16]. EBCT also offered sufficient resolution to adequately capture CAC in a moving heart. However, EBCT was inadequate for general CT imaging and was replaced by modern multidetector computed tomographic scanners (MDCT). Gantry rotation generates a cross-sectional image of the heart by taking several thousand pictures from different angels [17]. This creates a high definition image of the heart including coronary arteries. Most scans are executed with 0.5–1.5 mSv of radiation (similar to 10 chest X-Rays) [1].

CAC scans are executed with non-contrast, cardiac gated CT scanners. CAC is visible in unenhanced images, as calcified deposits in coronary arteries heavily attenuate X-rays [1]. Modern MDCTs with faster gantry rotations and more detector rows make CAC detection possible even in ungated MDCT scans. Even though ungated MDCT is not formally used for quantitative CAC scoring, evidence suggests that visual assessment of CAC in a non-gated routine chest CT accurately predicts Agatston score ranges (0, 1 to 100, 101 to 400, and >400) [18, 19]. Ungated MDCT are beneficial as they allow for the combination of CAC scoring as well as lung cancer screening [20]. The Society of Cardiovascular Computed Tomography (SCCT)/Society of Thoracic Radiology awarded a Class I recommendation for the evaluation of qualitative CAC scoring in non-contrast chest CT scans [21].

CAC Scoring

In general, the Agatston score is used to quantify CAC scans. The Agatston score is a sum of all calcified lesions of the coronary arteries through the z-axis of the heart, weighed by density of the calcium [22]. The score for an individual lesion is calculated by multiplying the lesion area with the density weighting factor (DWF), which originates from the greatest attenuation within the calcified lesion [23]. The individual Agatston score of all lesions in all coronary arteries are summed to obtain the total Agatston score [23] (Fig. 2). Other scoring methods include the volume score, which is highly similar to the Agatston score but does not rely on lesion density but instead calculates the lesion volume by multiplying the number of voxels by the volume of each voxel [23]. Currently, the Agatston score is seen as the gold standard of CAC scoring due to its simplicity, as well as being the first scoring method developed. However, the ideal CAC score is still being debated as critiques argue it is lacking in many respects. Potential improvements may stem from accounting for the regional distribution of calcium and extra-coronary calcification, as well as differential calculations of calcium density [23] (Fig. 3). Implementation of characteristics like calcium volume, density and plaque features into CAC calculators could improve risk discrimination for younger and older individuals whose particular risk characteristics are not optimally accounted for in traditional models [23, 24].

Early Data

A range of early, small studies investigated the relationship between CAC and detection of obstructive coronary artery disease (CAD). Here, CAC burden correlated with atherosclerotic plaque and CAC scoring was highly sensitive for CAD and associated with a very high negative predictive value [25–29].

However, understanding of CAC quickly shifted from detection of obstructive CAD to one of quantification of plaque burden. For instance, Sangiogri et al. demonstrated in a histopathological study a significant relation between plaque area and CAC, but no association between CAC and lumen area [30]. In another histopathological study examining coronary arteries from autopsy hearts, Rumberger et al. demonstrated that CAC and coronary artery plaque areas were highly correlated for whole hearts, individual coronary arteries as well as for segments of coronary arteries [31]. The strong risk-predictive value of CAC was also established early on by smaller studies. For instance, data on 4,903 asymptomatic patients in the St. Francis Heart study after 4.3 years of follow up demonstrated that

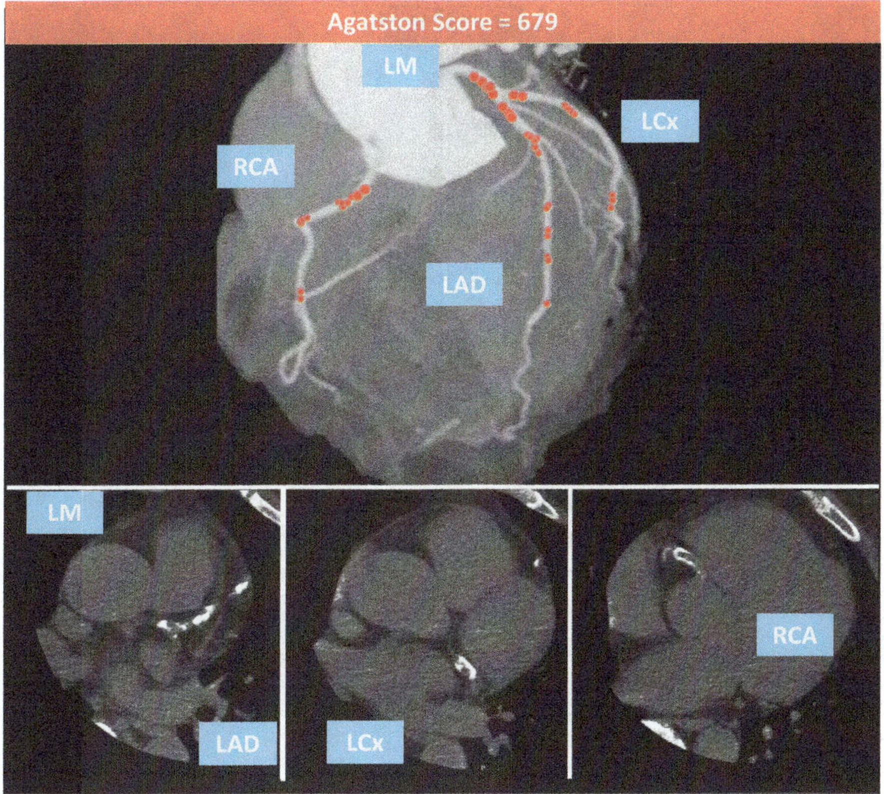

Fig. 2 Adapted *from CAC-DRS: Coronary Artery Calcium Data and Reporting System. An expert consensus document of the Society of Cardiovascular Computed Tomography (SCCT),* 2018, Journal of Cardiovascular Computed Tomography. Agatston score example. CAC=coronary artery calcium; LAD = left anterior descending; LCx = left circumflex; LM = left main; RCA = right coronary artery

CAC predicted CAD events independent of standard risk factors and was superior to the Framingham risk score (area under the curve (AUC) 0.79 vs. 0.69) [32]. More publications elucidated the positive risk predictive value of CAC for specific subpopulations, such as patients with diabetes [33], smokers [34], as well as elderly and young individuals [35].

Major Population-Based Studies

Major population-based studies established CAC as an effective tool for facilitating patient risk estimation and guiding primary preventive therapy decisions.

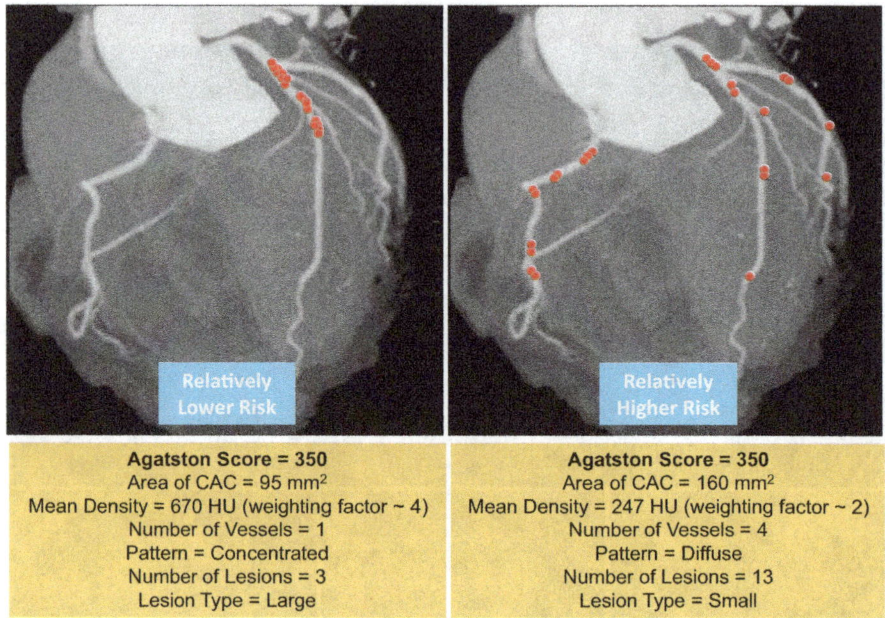

Fig. 3 Adapted from Blaha et al. *Coronary Artery Calcium Scoring Is It Time for a Change in Methodology?*, 2017, JACC Imaging. Both scans have an Agatston CAC score of 350. However, CAC area, density, distribution of CAC, number of calcified lesions and average lesion size differ in the scans. CAC=coronary artery calcium

MESA

The Multi-Ethnic Study of Atherosclerosis (MESA) investigated the prevalence, correlation and progression of subclinical CVD in 6,814 individuals belonging to four ethnicities (White, African-American, Hispanic, and Chinese). In a series of pioneering publications, MESA demonstrated that multiple markers of subclinical CVD improved coronary heart disease (CHD) risk prediction when added to traditional Framingham risk factors [36]. CAC was shown to have the greatest enhancement in prognostic capabilities of all risk factors. In the first landmark MESA publication, Detrano et al. reported the relationship between CAC and CHD. CAC provided predictive information over traditional risk factors with similar strength in all 4 ethnicities [37]. The authors also established that the addition of CAC to traditional risk models improves risk prediction more than any other test or traditional risk factors. The AUC for prediction of major coronary events as well as any coronary event was greater when CAC was added to standard risk factors (0.79 to 0.83 (p = 0.006) and 0.77 to 0.82 (p < 0.001)) [37]. Different CAC distributions were noted between ethnicities, with higher CAC prevalence in whites compared with the three other ethnic groups [38]. Compared to a CAC score of 0, a CAC score 1–100 was associated with a nearly fourfold higher risk of coronary event

(95% confidence interval (CI) 1.72–8.79) in multi-variable adjusted models and a CAC score > 300 was even associated with a sevenfold higher ASCVD event risk (95% CI 2.93–15.99) [37]. Doubling of CAC score was associated with a 15–35% increase in risk for major coronary event (95% CI 1.12–1.29) [37]. To further solidify these results, Polonsky et al. calculated the net reclassification improvement (NRI)—an index that attempts to quantify how well a new model reclassifies subjects as compared to an old model—before and after addition of CAC to traditional Framingham risk factors [39]. Addition of CAC resulted in 728 individuals being reclassified to a higher risk category and 814 to a lower risk factory. The overall NRI was 0.25 (95% CI 0.16–0.34).

Heinz Nixdorf

The population-based cohort Heinz Nixdorf Recall (HNR) study included 4,487 people from German cities between 45 and 75 years of age. 100% of men and 82% of women with known CAD had a CAC >0. HNR demonstrated similar results to MESA. For individuals deemed intermediate risk by Framingham risk factors, CAC testing reclassified 21.7% of individuals with CAC <100 into a lower risk group and 30.6% with CAC ≥ 400 into the high-risk category [40]. A CAC score of 0 was associated with an extremely low event rate of 0.16%/year. In contrast, participants with very high CAC scores had a 9–16 fold higher hazard ratio (HR) of ASCVD events than individuals without detectable CAC [41]. After adding CAC to the Framingham risk calculator, the AUC significantly increased from 0.681 to 0.749 (p = 0.003).

Rotterdam Study

The Rotterdam study was a prospective cohort study with 7,839 individuals in Rotterdam, Netherlands and included participants of older age (69.6 ± 6.2 years) than in MESA or HNR [42]. In all risk categories, the addition of CAC to Framingham risk model correctly reclassified 10-year risk of hard CHD events (NRI 0.14, p < 0.01). The largest share of reclassified individuals was observed in the intermediate Framingham risk group, in which 51% of men and 53% of women were reclassified.

Meta-Analysis

Due to the similarity of MESA, HNR and the Rotterdam Study, multiple meta analyses examined the predictive ability of CAC for specific subpopulations. Among 6739 women with low ASCVD risk from 5 cohort studies, CAC was present in approximately one-third of participants. The presence of CAC > 0 compared to a CAC score of 0 was associated with a significant increase in risk of

ASCVD events (HR 2.04 (95% CI 1.44–2.90)) [43]. A meta-analysis including the cohorts of three US studies (MESA, the Framingham Heart Study, Cardiovascular Health study) as well as two European cohorts (Rotterdam Study and HNR) examined the predictive ability of CAC score versus age for ASCVD risk prediction in elderly patients [44]. One third of participants had a CAC score of 0, which was associated with a low ASCVD event rate [44]. In the three US cohorts, CAC resulted in a more accurate reclassification of ASCVD risk than age. This was also the case in both European cohorts.

CAC in Guidelines

The CAC score as a risk prediction tool was noted in the 2013 ACC/AHA guidelines among a variety of other potential tests. In the current 2018 ACC/AHA cholesterol management guidelines and 2019 ACC/AHA primary prevention guidelines, the CAC score is recommended for asymptomatic individuals in the borderline and intermediate 10-year ASCVD risk group (5–20%) where risk estimates are uncertain. In very high (>20%) or low risk (<5%) risk patients, CAC scoring is not warranted because it does not meaningfully alter risk prediction in this group [45] (Fig. 4 and Table 1).

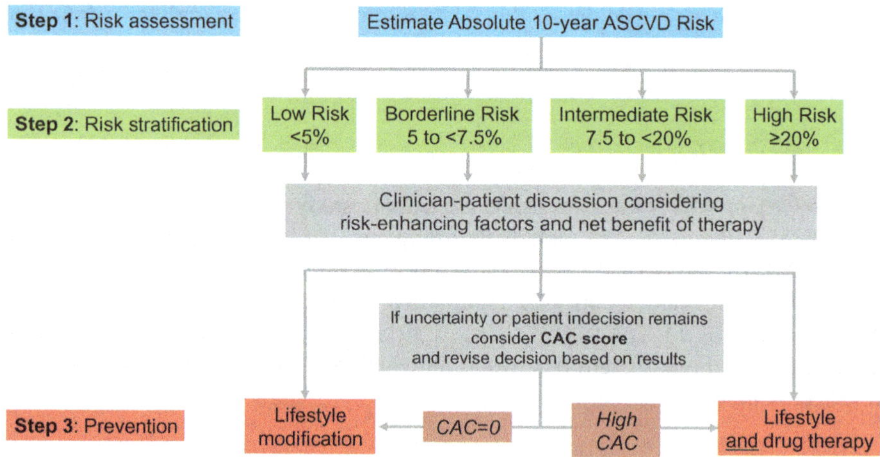

Fig. 4 Adapted from *2019 ACC/AHA Guideline on the Primary Prevention of Cardiovascular Disease.* For patients with borderline and intermediate risk, CAC scoring can individualize risk assessment and guide therapy decisions. ASCVD = Atherosclerotic cardiovascular disease; CAC=coronary artery calcium

Table 1 Primary preventive treatment by CAC score according to ACC/AHA 2018 guidelines

CAC score	Therapeutic consequence
CAC = 0	– In adults 40–75 years and LDL-C 70–189 mg/dL and intermediate risk (10 year ASCVD risk 7.5–19.9%) withhold statin therapy if no high risk conditions (diabetes mellitus, family history of premature CHD, cigarette smoking) – Avoid statins in older adults 76–80 years of age with LDL-C 70–189 mg/dL
CAC 1–99	– In adults 40–75 years and LDL-C 70–189 mg/dL and intermediate risk, initiate statin therapy if patient is ≥ 55 years of age
CAC > 100	In adults 40–75 years and LDL-C 70–189 mg/dL initiate statin therapy

ACC/AHA = American College of Cardiology/American Heart Association; ASCVD=atherosclerotic cardiovascular disease; CAC= coronary artery calcium; CHD = coronary heart disease; LDL-C = low-density lipoprotein cholesterol

Shared Decision-Making

2019 ACC/AHA primary prevention guidelines as well as the 2017 USPSTF are placing more emphasis on taking patient preferences into consideration. As discussed in more detail in Chapter 9 on Shared Decision Making, guidelines endorse a collaborative approach between clinicians and patients to decide on preventive therapy strategies [5, 21]. In a shared-decision making discussion, health care professionals should communicate the most recent evidence regarding risk assessment and preventive therapeutics, while allowing patients to express their preferences and values [5, 21, 46]. A risk discussion is particularly relevant to intermediate risk patients, as here risk-based decisions are often unclear and appropriate choices require a detailed understanding of ASCVD risk. Current guidelines recommend individualizing risk decisions by assessing risk enhancing factors as well as CAC after initial risk assessment with PCE. Compared to risk enhancers such as family history of ASCVD as well as biomarkers like ankle-brachial index (ABI), high sensitivity C-reactive protein (hsCRP), CAC was the most effective marker to reclassify risk [47–49]. Visualization of cardiovascular risk through the CAC score also provides a tangible understanding of ASCVD for patients, facilitating risk discussions and enhancing therapy adherence [21]. Evidence suggests that knowledge of CAC can promote lifestyle and behavioral changes in asymptomatic individuals [50].

Risk Re-Classification Through CAC

Multiple publications showed that CAC consistently outperforms other biomarkers in the ability to further stratify ASCVD risk [45, 47]. The NRI for CAC was 0.66, compared to 0.02–0.1 for other biomarkers [49]. CAC could reclassify cardiovascular risk of about 50% of individuals and thereby prevent preventive medication initiation in patients initially eligible for statin therapy by 2013 ACC/AHA guidelines. Data from MESA demonstrated that patients with CAC >300 but without risk factors had a 3.5 times higher ASCVD event rate than individuals with > 3 traditional risk factors but a CAC score of 0 [51]. Even asymptomatic adults with minimal CAC (1–10) had a 3-times higher risk of CHD events than individuals without CAC [52].

For the first time, current guidelines more clearly recognize the potency of a CAC score of 0. When comparing 13 risk markers with data from the MESA study, CAC was the biomarker associated with the strongest downward classification of ASCVD risk [47]. A CAC score of 0 is associated with a low event and mortality rate (<1%) [53]. In a IIa recommendation, the guidelines state that statin therapy as primary preventive therapy can be withheld, at least as the initial strategy, in patients without high-risk conditions if CAC score = 0. However, a CAC score of 0 provides less reassurance in individuals with diabetes [54] or smokers [34] and the decision on preventive therapy should be made with other clinical information [1].

CAC Future Directions

CAC Score = 0

While extensive evidence has established that CAC = 0 is associated with an excellent prognosis, multiple questions regarding CAC = 0 need to be addressed in the future. For one, the warranty period of a CAC = 0 is not entirely explored and adequate time intervals for rescanning remain unclear. Two recent MESA studies included 3,116 participants with baseline CAC = 0 and follow-up scans over 10 years after baseline showing a prevalence of CAC > 0, CAC > 10, and CAC > 100 of 53, 36, and 8% respectively at 10 years. Using a 25% testing yield (number needed to scan = 4), the estimated warranty period of CAC > 0 varied between 3 to 7 years depending on sex and race/ethnicity. Approximately 15% progressed to CAC > 10 in 5 to 8 years, while 10-year progression to CAC > 100 was rare. The presence of diabetes was associated with a significantly shorter warranty period, while family history and smoking had small effects. 19% of all 10-year coronary events occurred in CAC = 0 prior to performance of a subsequent scan at 3–5 years, while new detection of CAC > 0 preceded 55% of future events and identified individuals at threefold higher risk of coronary events [55, 56]. However, more precise information on the warranty period of CAC = 0 in other major population-based studies is called for, taking into consideration race/ethnicity and risk enhancing conditions like diabetes, smokers or family history of CHD.

CAC Predicting Non-CVD Outcomes

Optimally, in the future CAC scoring could be used as a synergistic tool to predict CVD but as well as non-cardiovascular outcomes. The discussion of CAC as a measure of "biological age" gives rise to the notion of using CAC as a risk marker for non-CVD, age related diseases such as cancers and neurodegenerative diseases like dementia. Risk of death from non-CVD causes are associated with high levels of CAC [57]. Conversely, CAC = 0 appears protective against CVD as well as non-CVD events [58]. Eventually multi-disease screening will become the norm, such as combining screening for sub-clinical lung disease and sub-clinical cardio-vascular disease with CAC scoring. Since cancer is the leading cause of death next to CVD, the association of CAC scoring and risk of cancer mortality is of special interest. A MESA analysis demonstrated that individuals with CAC > 400 had a significantly higher risk of cancer (HR 1.53, 95% CI 1.18–1.99), compared to those with CAC = 0 [58]. Overall, future guidelines will likely embrace the possibility of predicting multiple ASCVD and non-CVD disease outcomes after CAC scanning.

Risk Estimators Incorporating CAC Scores

Currently there is only one existing risk calculator which includes CAC. The MESA-CHD risk score published in 2015 was the first risk calculator in which users had the option to calculate risk with integration of the CAC score [59]. With the use of 10-year of follow up data from MESA, McClelland et al. created a CHD risk score incorporating traditional risk factors as well as CAC information. The MESA risk calculator was validated by the Dallas Heart Study (DHS) and the HNR study. The external validation by the HNR established excellent calibration and discrimination [17]. Available online or per smartphone, users enter information on age, sex, race/ethnicity, traditional Framingham risk factors, family history of CHD and CAC score to calculate the 10-year risk of CHD with and without incorporation of CAC data. Risk calculators available for clinicians as well as patient use would help communicate cardiovascular risk to patients and be a helpful tool in shared decision-making discussions between clinicians and patients.

Coronary Computed Tomography Angiography

Technology

Coronary computed tomography angiography (CCTA) is performed by a multi-detector CT system and unlike CAC scanning, requires injection of iodine contrast. The final image is formed through a series of axial slices covering the entire length of the heart. With modern scanners, CCTA can be executed with radiation of 1–5 mSV, which of now is still higher than the 0.5–1.5mSV associated with CAC scans. Beta blockers are often administered prior to scanning, in order to limit radiation exposure and motion artifacts [60]. Isotropic voxels allow for 3D reconstruction of plaques.

Characterization of Atherosclerotic Plaque

The CAC score is a widely available, inexpensive, and simple test for quantifying atherosclerosis burden. However, this marker is not sufficient to gain full information regarding coronary plaque morphology. The native CT scan to obtain the CAC score only avails to diagnose calcified plaques and cannot detect the presence or extent of mixed or non-calcified plaques or their associated degree of luminal stenosis. The clinical importance of detecting non-calcified plaques is currently being debated. A study observed that individuals with low CAC score ($\leq$ 100) had a high prevalence of non-calcified plaques (83.3%) [61]. Non-calcified plaques are thought of as higher risk for plaque rupture, subsequently causing serious cardiac events. Stable plaques are causal to coronary artery stenosis, and are predominantly made up of calcified or mixed plaques [62]. However, according to multiple studies the prevalence of exclusively non-calcified plaques in patient populations is low. One publication suggested that 1–2% of symptomatic patients with angina and a CAC score of 0 have non-calcified CAD [63, 64]. These findings were not associated with future coronary revascularization or adverse prognosis within 2 years [63]. The COroNary CT Angiography Evaluation For Clinical Outcomes: An InteRnational Multicenter Registry (CONFIRM) registry study including 10,037 patients showed that only 3.5% of patients had obstructive CAD with a CAC score of 0. These patients did not have an elevated risk of all-cause mortality [65].

In addition to detecting the degree of calcification, CCTA was shown to identify characteristics atherosclerotic lesions most vulnerable for development of acute coronary syndrome (ACS) [66]. Data from the Prospective Multicenter Imaging Study for Evaluation of Chest Pain (PROMISE) study demonstrated that high-risk plaque detected by CCTA (positive remodeling, low CT attenuation or napkin ring sign) was significantly associated with major adverse cardiovascular events (MACE) (HR 1.73, 95% CI 1.13–2.26) [67]. Ferencik et al. similarly established that CT-based plaque morphology, such as positive remodeling, spotty calcium, stenosis length, low attenuation plaque volume provided high discriminatory value for detection of ACS in patients with acute chest pain [68].

Scoring/Measuring

SCCT guidelines recommend a simple approach for describing plaque types in CCTA [69]. All 17 coronary segments are visually classified by stenosis severity and plaque type. According to relative amounts of calcification, plaques are categorized into three categories: non-calcified, mixed plaque or calcified plaque.

Evidence for Clinical Outcome

The CONFIRM registry demonstrated that plaque burden and stenosis measured by CCTA carry significant prognostic value. A prognostic score using CCTA parameters improved risk prediction compared to traditional clinical risk scores [70].

Much evidence suggests the benefit of CAC severity visualized by CCTA as a treatment guide. In a very recent publication, Mortensen et al. modeled to what extent information of severity of CAD and LDL-C levels can benefit patients treating LDL-C to guideline targets. The authors calculated the NNT in 6 years to prevent 1 ASCVD event and the number of events prevented if LDL-C was treated to target and concluded that CCTA test results could individualize preventive treatment and identify patients who would benefit the most from lipid-lowering therapy. For example, the NNT in 6 years to prevent 1 ASCVD event by treating LDL-C to the ESC guidelines target was 8 for patients with 3-vessel CAD compared to 233 for patients with no CAD assessed by CCTA [71].

Multiple large, randomized-controlled trials provide evidence of improved clinical outcome after using CCTA. PROMISE, a large cohort study enrolling 10,003 patients, assessed the clinical outcome of patients assigned to anatomical testing with CCTA compared to functional testing. While the PROMISE study had a neutral outcome for the primary endpoint of death, myocardial infarction, hospitalization for unstable angina or major procedural complications after 2 years of follow up, the authors did report a 34% relative reduction in all-cause death and myocardial infarction at 12 months for those receiving CCTA [72].

The Scottish Computed Tomography of the Heart (SCOT-HEART) Trial recruited patients aged 18–75 years who had been referred to a cardiology clinic from their primary physician for suspected stable angina from CHD [73]. Patients were randomized to standard care plus CAC and CCTA, or standard care alone. Standard care included routine examination and if appropriate, stress test and invasive coronary angiography. The SCOT-HEART trial demonstrated a clear reduction in the composite long-term endpoint of coronary heart disease after 5 years for patients who underwent CCTA compared to standard care alone (HR 0.59, 95% CI 0.41–0.84; p = 0.004) [73].

Authors of the Computed Tomography versus Exercise Testing in Suspected Coronary Artery Disease (CRESCENT) randomized controlled trial compared the efficacy of a tiered cardiac CT protocol based on calcium imaging with functional testing. Here, for patients with suspected stable CAD, a tiered cardiac CT protocol offered an effective and safe alternative to functional testing. Incorporating the calcium scan into the diagnostic workup was safe and lowered radiation exposure. After 1 year, CT scanning was cost effective, reducing overall diagnostic costs by 16% [74]. Even though underpowered for clinical events, CRESCENT demonstrated a lower rate of myocardial infarctions in patients diagnosed with CCTA [74]. Plank et al. demonstrated that coronary plaque burden identified by CCTA was associated with MACE. Patients with SIS $>$ = 5 (Coronary segment involvement score, total number of segments with plaque) had a HR of 6.5 (95% CI 1.6–25.8, p < 0.013) for MACE [75].

However, the use of routine CCTA as a screening modality for high-risk asymptomatic groups was not beneficial. In FACTOR-64, routine screening for CAD in patients with type 1 and type 2 diabetes mellitus and CCTA directed therapy did not reduce risk of death or coronary outcomes [76].

CCTA Versus CAC

At present, CCTA is most useful to rule out CAD in high-risk, symptomatic patients with known or suspected CHD. (Fig. 5) The added benefit of relying on CCTA beyond CAC for asymptomatic patients has not yet been confirmed. The key question remains how the prognostic information from less conclusive CCTA could be deciphered—especially in those with extensive CAC—and, at the same time, improve the pre-test probability accrued to better select patients who need to undergo further imaging testing. Results from an observational registry including 27,125 patients compared the predictive value of CCTA and CAC to diagnose CAD in patients without chest pain syndrome [77]. While both imaging modalities improved the performance of standard risk factor prediction models for all-cause mortality and the composite outcome (all-cause mortality and nonfatal myocardial infarction), CAC scoring provided greater incremental discriminatory value than CCTA [77]. The large randomized clinical trial, SCOT-HEART II, will assess whether cardiovascular outcomes are improved with CCTA screening compared to standard of care in asymptomatic patients.

Extra-Coronary Atherosclerosis Imaging

Carotid Artery Ultrasound

Ultrasound can non-invasively measure the carotid vessel wall, and historically B-mode ultrasound has been used to measure the thickness of the intima-media layer of the vessel wall (carotid intima media thickness (CIMT)). CIMT is an established measure of an arteriosclerosis-like process, and multiple studies have demonstrated a positive association between increased CIMT and degree of atherosclerosis identified by invasive angiography [78–80]. Indeed the cellular and molecular mechanisms underlying early atherosclerosis lead to intima-media thickening. However, carotid wall thickening is not completely synonymous with atherosclerosis, as CIMT increases with advancing age and hypertension induced media thickening [81, 82].

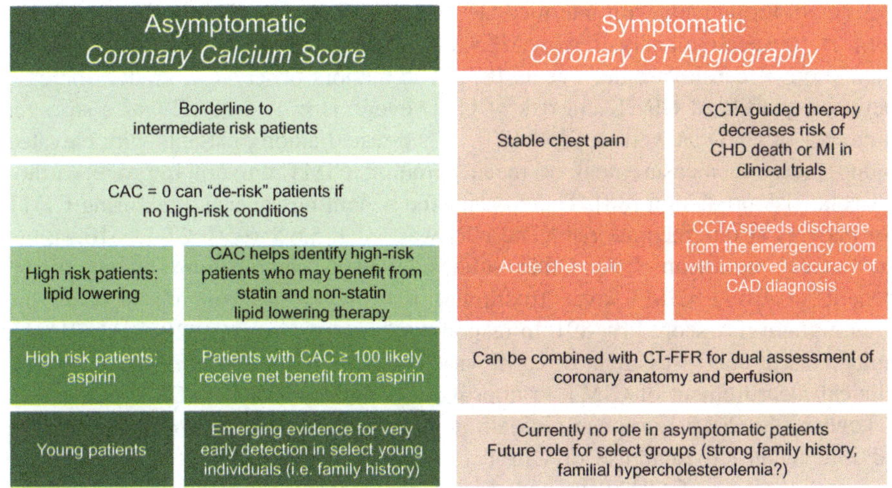

Fig. 5 Emerging consensuses for use of CT in precision medicine adapted from Cardoso et al. Cardiac Computed Tomography for Personalized Management of Patients with Type 2 Diabetes Mellitus 2020, Circulation: Cardiovascular Imaging. Overview of coronary artery calcium (CAC) and coronary computed tomography angiography (CCTA) in the evaluation of asymptomatic and symptomatic patients. CAC=coronary artery calcium; CAD = coronary artery disease; CCTA = coronary computed tomography angiography; CHD = coronary heart disease; CT-FFR = computed tomography angiography derived-fractional flow reserve; MI = myocardial infarction

Ultrasound Carotid Plaque Imaging

Ultrasound measures of carotid plaque on the other hand is distinctive to advanced stages of atherosclerosis, as it is a result of atherogenic lipoprotein entry into the arterial wall, followed by inflammation, oxidative stress and endothelial cell dysfunction [83]. The American Society of Echocardiography recommends to quantify atherosclerotic plaque in the common carotid artery, carotid bifurcation, and internal carotid artery [84]. While CIMT is most easily measured in the common carotid artery due to its perpendicular location to the ultrasound beam, atherosclerotic plaque most often occurs downstream in the outer wall of carotid artery bulb, which is not as accurately measured by CIMT. A meta-analysis demonstrated that the ultrasound assessment of carotid plaque had a higher diagnostic accuracy for the prediction of CAD and future myocardial infarcts than CIMT measures alone [85].

These factors may explain the limited improvement of traditional risk assessment with CIMT. The benefit of adding CIMT measurements to the traditional Framingham risk score was evaluated in a meta-analysis including 45,828 individuals of 14 cohort studies [86]. Incorporation of CIMT resulted in a small improvement in 10-year risk prediction (NRI 0.8%; 95% CI 0.1–1.6) [86]. Albeit still small, for patients with intermediate risk, the NRI was a slightly higher at 3.6% [86]. A prospective analysis with MESA data compared CIMT to CAC score for prediction of cardiovascular events [87]. The authors observed a graded increase between quartile of CIMT and risk of CVD event. However, CAC was a stronger predictor of CHD as well as CVD [87]. When tested among patients with elevated blood pressure, measurement of mean common CIMT did not improve cardio-vascular risk prediction [88]. There was some benefit however in measuring CIMT for patients at intermediate risk. The NRI was small 5.6% (95% CI 1.6–10.4), but statistically significant [88]. Other studies failed to demonstrate any significant benefit of using CIMT over traditional risk factor assessment, such as the Framingham risk score [49, 89]. In response to this evidence, the 2013 ACC/AHA guidelines on the assessment of cardiovascular risk do not recommend the routine clinical measurement of CIMT to improve risk assessment of ASCVD events [3]. Likewise, the 2016 European Guidelines on CVD prevention in clinical practice advised against regular use of CIMT for risk stratification [90]. Some evidence suggests the use of CIMT in pediatric patients. Part of the appeal stems from CIMT's non-invasive nature, lack of side effects as well as the ability to detect subclinical disease prior to symptoms. Multiple studies observed an association between CIMT and exposure to parental cardiovascular risk enhancers, such as smoking and maternal high blood pressure, in children 5 years of age [91, 92].

CT-Detected Extra-Coronary Atherosclerosis

Detection of extra-coronary calcification (ECC) has been discussed as possibly improving ASCVD risk prediction. Atherosclerosis is a systemic process, thus measuring calcification of multiple sites into consideration may be more repre-sentative of the diffuse nature of whole-body atherosclerosis [93]. Even though currently measuring the calcification burden outside of the coronary arteries does not predict ASCVD events better than CAC, ECC has the advantage of being identifiable on multiple imaging modalities like radiography, echocardiography, ultrasound and routine chest CTs [94–96]. Thus, information on atherosclerotic burden can be obtained without additional cost or radiation exposure. Using MESA data, Tison et al. evaluated the prognostic value of multi-site ECC for CHD events, CHD mortality and all-cause mortality [93]. The results suggest that ECC is highly prevalent (45% of patients). Patients with detectable ECC in 4 sites had a two-fold higher risk of outcomes independent of CAC score.

Magnetic Resonance Imaging

Due to the soft tissue contrast, magnetic resonance imaging (MRI) is well suited for atherosclerotic plaque visualization of large arteries. Unlike ultrasound, MRI can visualize plaque components specific to vulnerable plaque that are more prone to rupture [97]. Accurate identification of vulnerable plaques is significant, as 60–70% of acute MIs and almost all of ischemic strokes are caused by plaque rupture [98, 99]. In a meta-analysis of 8 studies with 690 participants, the presence of carotid intra-plaque hemorrhage identified by MRI was associated with a sixfold higher risk of cerebrovascular events [100]. The detection of vulnerable plaque may also inform status of atherosclerosis disease in other vessels, as certain plaque phenotypes are associated with events from coronary arteries [101]. In a MESA study, adverse carotid arterial remodeling and lipid core identified by MRI was associated with an increased risk of cardiovascular events in asymptomatic subjects [102]. However, carotid MRI is still considered a specialty technique that is time consuming and costly, thus it is not considered a viable option for population risk assessment.

Tests for Myocardial Ischemia

Single photon emission computed tomography and positron emission tomography myocardial perfusion imaging.

Single photon emission computed tomography (SPECT) is used for visualizing myocardial perfusion as a result of coronary blood flow while positron emission tomography (PET) myocardial perfusion imaging (MPI) further enables quantification of myocardial perfusion. The unifying principle of these two imaging modalities is that a contrast medium is given via a peripheral vein, which then circulates in the body, enabling visualization of the perfusion of all myocardial tissue at both rest and stress. These tests can identify patients with reduced coronary blood flow or coronary blood flow reserve, which is often the result of obstructive CAD but can also be caused by non-obstructive CAC or other conditions such as coronary vasospasm.

In addition, radioactive tracers have been developed which accumulate in areas where pathological processes specific to cardiovascular disease is occurring. In the PET scan, early atherosclerosis can be detected by using 18-fluoro-deoxyglucose (FDG) as a tracer. Enhanced FDG uptake is a sign of vascular inflammation and thereby visualizes early manifestations of atherosclerosis. More specific tracers such as 18-F-NaF or 68-Ga-DOTATATE are characterized by low uptake in the myocardium and are therefore better suited for detecting plaque in the coronary arteries [103, 104]. Similar tracers for inflammation imaging have been developed for SPECT.

SPECT and PET MPI are highly accurate for diagnosis of obstructive CAD. A study of 7,061 patients demonstrated that the severity of ischemia and scar as detected by PET MPI significantly improved risk reclassification of cardiac death (NRI 0.116 (95% CI 0.021–0.210)) [105]. A smaller study by Yoshinaga et al. evaluated the prognostic capabilities of stress PET MPI with rubidium-82 (^{82}RB) for cardiac events. A normal stress ^{82}RB PET MPI was associated with an excellent prognosis, with an annual hard cardiac event rate of 0.4% [106]. However, routine screening for CAD with PET MPI did not significantly improve outcomes among high risk patients. Type 2 diabetes patients in the Detection of Ischemia in Asymptomatic Diabetics (DIAD) study did not have significantly lower rates of cardiac death or nonfatal myocardial infarction when screened with PET MPI for myocardial ischemia [107]. However, one major limitation of PET MPI imaging is that it is unable to identify nonobstructive CAD, as MPI can only visualize reduced blood flow, which is a late finding in ASCVD. Studies have shown that patients with normal SPECT results and subsequent CAC scanning, had evidence of atherosclerosis, often with severe CAC scores [108]. The synergistic use between CAC scoring and PET MPI may overcome this limitation and improve diagnostic accuracy [109]. Engbers et al. evaluated this approach by referring 4,897 asymptomatic patients to stress-rest SPECT-MPI and CAC scoring. The authors observed a step-wise increase in adverse cardiac events with increasing CAC scores and SPECT-MPI abnormalities. In asymptomatic patients with high CAC score (CAC > 400), SPECT is considered "appropriate" [110]. It was demonstrated that frequency of myocardial ischemia increased with increasing CAC score [108]. In high-risk patients, SPECT-MPI imaging may be warranted earlier at a lower CAC threshold. For instance, among patients with CAC score 100–399, 13.0% of diabetic individuals had frequent ischemia's compared to 2.3% of non-diabetics [111].

Structural Imaging

Echocardiography

Resting transthoracic echocardiography using ultrasound provides a detailed view of cardiac chambers, valves, and function and is broadly used to assess patients with structural heart disease or suspicious symptoms. However, echocardiography does not have the spatial resolution nor does ultrasound have the penetrance to detect atherosclerosis of the coronaries. Population-based studies on asymptomatic individuals found that incidental diagnosis of left ventricular (LV) dysfunction and LV hypertrophy with echocardiography is associated with cardiovascular and all-cause mortality and was independent of blood pressure and other risk factors [112]. In response, the 2010 American College of Cardiology Foundation and the American Heart Association (ACCF/AHA) guidelines awarded a weak recommendation (class IIb recommendation) for echocardiography screening for LV hypertrophy and LV dysfunction in asymptomatic adults with hypertension [112, 113]. However, widespread screening with echocardiography is not recommended, and is in fact discouraged. Meaningful abnormalities in the healthy population are rare, echocardiography is not specific to ASCVD, and therefore it adds little to risk assessment in a general population.

Cardiac Magnetic Resonance

While echocardiography is used more often in the clinical setting for routine assessment of cardiac structure and function, cardiac magnetic resonance (CMR) is more reproduceable and accurate. With the application of contrast, myocardial scar tissue and fibrosis can be visualized. In addition, CMR can effectively measure LV size and function. Results from the Dallas Heart Study suggested strong association between LV hypertrophy measured by CMR and risk of adverse CV outcomes [114]. However, CMR does not have the spatial resolution for routine assessment of coronary atherosclerosis, and it is costly and image acquisition takes a long time. CMR can be used for detection of myocardial ischemia in stress testing protocols, however there is currently no role for CMR-guided risk assessment in the general healthy population.

Diagnostic Accuracy of Cardiac Imaging

Compared to traditional risk factors, cardiac imaging is much more sensitive for detection of early atherosclerosis compared to cardiovascular risk assessment with traditional risk-factors. Due to cardiac imaging's high sensitivity it is also associated with a high negative predictive value for ASCVD and thereby an excellent tool for downgrading low-risk patients [115]. CAC in particular is one of the most sensitive cardiac imaging modalities. For high-risk patients with a higher pre-test probability of CAD, imaging tests with a higher specificity such as CCTA are recommended. Thus, current consensus is using CAC as a gatekeeper to more invasive testing like CCTA in low-intermediate risk patients.

Conclusion

The promise of precision medicine is giving the right patient the right therapy at the right time based on their highly personal characteristics. In the field of risk prediction, consensus is moving toward direct detection of overall burden of atherosclerosis to create a personalized estimation of cardiovascular risk, instead of relying on a population-based 10-year risk estimate reliant on the number of traditional risk factors present. Also, these risk factors were measured commonly at a single point time, which is subject to measurement error and does not take into account the cumulative exposure. Cardiac imaging is a highly effective tool given its sensitivity for detecting a clinically important burden coronary atherosclerosis, along with its specificity in detecting atherosclerosis directly versus merely risk for atherosclerosis. Identifying patients with the highest risk of ASCVD who would benefit most of preventive treatment is paramount, as this would focus resources on risk reduction strategies in the right patients at the right time and avoid aggressive treatment in patients who are in fact low-risk. By determining an individual's distinctive CAD burden, cardiac imaging can facilitate personalized allocation of primary and secondary preventive therapy and improve ASCVD outcomes.

References

1. Michos ED, Blaha MJ, Martin SS, Blumenthal RS. 29—screening for atherosclerotic cardiovascular disease in asymptomatic individuals. In: de Lemos JA, Omland T, editors. Chronic Coronary Artery Disease. Elsevier; 2018. p. 459–78.
2. Force USPST. Using nontraditional risk factors in coronary heart disease risk assessment: U. S. Preventive Services Task Force recommendation statement. Ann Intern Med. 2009;151 (7):474–82. doi: https://doi.org/10.7326/0003-4819-151-7-200910060-00008.
3. Goff DC Jr, Lloyd-Jones DM, Bennett G, Coady S, D'Agostino RB, Gibbons R, et al. 2013 ACC/AHA guideline on the assessment of cardiovascular risk: a report of the American college of cardiology/American heart association task force on practice guidelines. Circulation. 2014;129(25 Suppl 2):S49-73. https://doi.org/10.1161/01.cir.0000437741. 48606.98.
4. Grundy SM, Stone NJ, Bailey AL, Beam C, Birtcher KK, Blumenthal RS, et al. 2018 AHA/ ACC/AACVPR/AAPA/ABC/ACPM/ADA/AGS/APhA/ASPC/NLA/PCNA guideline on the management of blood cholesterol: executive summary: a report of the American college of cardiology/American heart association task force on clinical practice guidelines. J Am Coll Cardiol. 2019;73(24):3168–209. https://doi.org/10.1016/j.jacc.2018.11.002.
5. Arnett DK, Blumenthal RS, Albert MA, Buroker AB, Goldberger ZD, Hahn EJ, et al. 2019 ACC/AHA guideline on the primary prevention of cardiovascular disease: a report of the American college of cardiology/American heart association task force on clinical practice guidelines. J Am Coll Cardiol. 2019;74(10):e177-232. https://doi.org/10.1016/j.jacc.2019. 03.010.
6. Shah AM, Claggett B, Loehr LR, Chang PP, Matsushita K, Kitzman D, et al. Heart failure stages among older adults in the community: the atherosclerosis risk in communities study. Circulation. 2017;135(3):224–40. https://doi.org/10.1161/CIRCULATIONAHA.116. 023361.
7. Yancy CW, Jessup M, Bozkurt B, Butler J, Casey DE Jr, Colvin MM, et al. 2017 ACC/ AHA/HFSA focused update of the 2013 ACCF/AHA guideline for the management of heart failure: a report of the American college of cardiology/American heart association task force on clinical practice guidelines and the heart failure society of America. Circulation. 2017;136(6):e137–61. https://doi.org/10.1161/CIR.0000000000000509.
8. Felker GM, Anstrom KJ, Adams KF, Ezekowitz JA, Fiuzat M, Houston-Miller N, et al. Effect of natriuretic peptide-guided therapy on hospitalization or cardiovascular mortality in high-risk patients with heart failure and reduced ejection fraction: a randomized clinical trial. JAMA. 2017;318(8):713–20. https://doi.org/10.1001/jama.2017.10565.
9. Stienen S, Salah K, Moons AH, Bakx AL, van Pol P, Kortz RAM, et al. NT-proBNP (N-Terminal pro-B-Type Natriuretic Peptide)-Guided therapy in acute decompensated heart failure: PRIMA II randomized controlled trial (Can NT-ProBNP-Guided Therapy During Hospital Admission for Acute Decompensated Heart Failure Reduce Mortality and Readmissions?). Circulation. 2018;137(16):1671–83. https://doi.org/10.1161/ CIRCULATIONAHA.117.029882.
10. Sabatine MS, Morrow DA, de Lemos JA, Omland T, Sloan S, Jarolim P, et al. Evaluation of multiple biomarkers of cardiovascular stress for risk prediction and guiding medical therapy

in patients with stable coronary disease. Circulation. 2012;125(2):233–40. https://doi.org/10. 1161/CIRCULATIONAHA.111.063842.

11. Wang TJ, Gona P, Larson MG, Tofler GH, Levy D, Newton-Cheh C, et al. Multiple biomarkers for the prediction of first major cardiovascular events and death. N Engl J Med. 2006;355(25):2631–9. https://doi.org/10.1056/NEJMoa055373.

12. Kim HC, Greenland P, Rossouw JE, Manson JE, Cochrane BB, Lasser NL, et al. Multimarker prediction of coronary heart disease risk: the Women's Health Initiative. J Am Coll Cardiol. 2010;55(19):2080–91. https://doi.org/10.1016/j.jacc.2009.12.047.

13. Kosmala W, Przewlocka-Kosmala M, Rojek A, Marwick TH. Comparison of the diastolic stress test with a combined resting echocardiography and biomarker approach to patients with exertional dyspnea: diagnostic and prognostic implications. JACC Cardiovasc Imaging. 2019;12(5):771–80. https://doi.org/10.1016/j.jcmg.2017.10.008.

14. Kalogeropoulos AP, Georgiopoulou VV, deFilippi CR, Gottdiener JS, Butler J, Cardiovascular HS. Echocardiography, natriuretic peptides, and risk for incident heart failure in older adults: the Cardiovascular Health Study. JACC Cardiovasc Imaging. 2012;5 (2):131–40. https://doi.org/10.1016/j.jcmg.2011.11.011.

15. Detrano R, Markovic D, Simpfendorfer C, Franco I, Hollman J, Grigera F, et al. Digital subtraction fluoroscopy: a new method of detecting coronary calcifications with improved sensitivity for the prediction of coronary disease. Circulation. 1985;71(4):725–32. https:// doi.org/10.1161/01.cir.71.4.725.

16. Agatston AS, Janowitz WR, Hildner FJ, Zusmer NR, Viamonte M Jr, Detrano R. Quantification of coronary artery calcium using ultrafast computed tomography. J Am Coll Cardiol. 1990;15(4):827–32. https://doi.org/10.1016/0735-1097(90)90282-t.

17. Greenland P, Blaha MJ, Budoff MJ, Erbel R, Watson KE. Coronary Calcium Score and Cardiovascular Risk. J Am Coll Cardiol. 2018;72(4):434–47. https://doi.org/10.1016/j.jacc. 2018.05.027.

18. Blair KJ, Allison MA, Morgan C, Wassel CL, Rifkin DE, Wright CM, et al. Comparison of ordinal versus Agatston coronary calcification scoring for cardiovascular disease mortality in community-living individuals. Int J Cardiovasc Imaging. 2014;30(4):813–8. https://doi.org/ 10.1007/s10554-014-0392-1.

19. Azour L, Kadoch MA, Ward TJ, Eber CD, Jacobi AH. Estimation of cardiovascular risk on routine chest CT: ordinal coronary artery calcium scoring as an accurate predictor of Agatston score ranges. J Cardiovasc Comput Tomogr. 2017;11(1):8–15. https://doi.org/10. 1016/j.jcct.2016.10.001.

20. Budoff MJ, Nasir K, Kinney GL, Hokanson JE, Barr RG, Steiner R, et al. Coronary artery and thoracic calcium on noncontrast thoracic CT scans: comparison of ungated and gated examinations in patients from the COPD Gene cohort. J Cardiovasc Comput Tomogr. 2011;5(2):113–8. https://doi.org/10.1016/j.jcct.2010.11.002.

21. Hecht H, Blaha MJ, Berman DS, Nasir K, Budoff M, Leipsic J, et al. Clinical indications for coronary artery calcium scoring in asymptomatic patients: expert consensus statement from the society of cardiovascular computed tomography. J Cardiovasc Comput Tomogr. 2017;11 (2):157–68. https://doi.org/10.1016/j.jcct.2017.02.010.

22. Alluri K, Joshi PH, Henry TS, Blumenthal RS, Nasir K, Blaha MJ. Scoring of coronary artery calcium scans: history, assumptions, current limitations, and future directions. Atherosclerosis. 2015;239(1):109–17. https://doi.org/10.1016/j.atherosclerosis.2014.12.040.

23. Blaha MJ, Mortensen MB, Kianoush S, Tota-Maharaj R, Cainzos-Achirica M. Coronary artery calcium scoring: is it time for a change in methodology? JACC Cardiovasc Imaging. 2017;10(8):923–37. https://doi.org/10.1016/j.jcmg.2017.05.007.

24. Criqui MH, Denenberg JO, Ix JH, McClelland RL, Wassel CL, Rifkin DE, et al. Calcium density of coronary artery plaque and risk of incident cardiovascular events. JAMA. 2014;311(3):271–8. https://doi.org/10.1001/jama.2013.282535.

25. Rumberger JA, Schwartz RS, Simons DB, Sheedy PF 3rd, Edwards WD, Fitzpatrick LA. Relation of coronary calcium determined by electron beam computed tomography and

lumen narrowing determined by autopsy. Am J Cardiol. 1994;73(16):1169–73. https://doi. org/10.1016/0002-9149(94)90176-7.

26. Margolis JR, Chen JT, Kong Y, Peter RH, Behar VS, Kisslo JA. The diagnostic and prognostic significance of coronary artery calcification. A report of 800 cases. Radiology. 1980;137(3):609–16. doi: https://doi.org/10.1148/radiology.137.3.7444045.

27. Shavelle DM, Budoff MJ, LaMont DH, Shavelle RM, Kennedy JM, Brundage BH. Exercise testing and electron beam computed tomography in the evaluation of coronary artery disease. J Am Coll Cardiol. 2000;36(1):32–8. https://doi.org/10.1016/s0735-1097(00)00696-3.

28. Budoff MJ, Diamond GA, Raggi P, Arad Y, Guerci AD, Callister TQ, et al. Continuous probabilistic prediction of angiographically significant coronary artery disease using electron beam tomography. Circulation. 2002;105(15):1791–6. https://doi.org/10.1161/01.cir. 0000014483.43921.8c.

29. Simons DB, Schwartz RS, Edwards WD, Sheedy PF, Breen JF, Rumberger JA. Noninvasive definition of anatomic coronary artery disease by ultrafast computed tomographic scanning: a quantitative pathologic comparison study. J Am Coll Cardiol. 1992;20(5):1118–26. https:// doi.org/10.1016/0735-1097(92)90367-v.

30. Sangiorgi G, Rumberger JA, Severson A, Edwards WD, Gregoire J, Fitzpatrick LA, et al. Arterial calcification and not lumen stenosis is highly correlated with atherosclerotic plaque burden in humans: a histologic study of 723 coronary artery segments using nondecalcifying methodology. J Am Coll Cardiol. 1998;31(1):126–33. https://doi.org/10.1016/s0735-1097 (97)00443-9.

31. Rumberger JA, Simons DB, Fitzpatrick LA, Sheedy PF, Schwartz RS. Coronary artery calcium area by electron-beam computed tomography and coronary atherosclerotic plaque area A histopathologic correlative study. Circulation. 1995;92(8):2157–62. https://doi.org/ 10.1161/01.cir.92.8.2157.

32. Arad Y, Goodman KJ, Roth M, Newstein D, Guerci AD. Coronary calcification, coronary disease risk factors, C-reactive protein, and atherosclerotic cardiovascular disease events: the St. Francis Heart Study. J Am Coll Cardiol. 2005;46(1):158–65. doi: https://doi.org/10.1016/ j.jacc.2005.02.088.

33. Raggi P, Shaw LJ, Berman DS, Callister TQ. Prognostic value of coronary artery calcium screening in subjects with and without diabetes. J Am Coll Cardiol. 2004;43(9):1663–9. https://doi.org/10.1016/j.jacc.2003.09.068.

34. McEvoy JW, Blaha MJ, Rivera JJ, Budoff MJ, Khan AN, Shaw LJ, et al. Mortality rates in smokers and nonsmokers in the presence or absence of coronary artery calcification. JACC Cardiovasc Imaging. 2012;5(10):1037–45. https://doi.org/10.1016/j.jcmg.2012.02.017.

35. Tota-Maharaj R, Blaha MJ, McEvoy JW, Blumenthal RS, Muse ED, Budoff MJ, et al. Coronary artery calcium for the prediction of mortality in young adults <45 years old and elderly adults >75 years old. Eur Heart J. 2012;33(23):2955–62. https://doi.org/10.1093/ eurheartj/ehs230.

36. Blaha MJ, Yeboah J, Al Rifai M, Liu K, Kronmal R, Greenland P. Providing evidence for subclinical CVD in risk assessment. Glob Heart. 2016;11(3):275–85. https://doi.org/10. 1016/j.gheart.2016.08.003.

37. Detrano R, Guerci AD, Carr JJ, Bild DE, Burke G, Folsom AR, et al. Coronary calcium as a predictor of coronary events in four racial or ethnic groups. N Engl J Med. 2008;358 (13):1336–45. https://doi.org/10.1056/NEJMoa072100.

38. McClelland RL, Chung H, Detrano R, Post W, Kronmal RA. Distribution of coronary artery calcium by race, gender, and age: results from the Multi-Ethnic Study of Atherosclerosis (MESA). Circulation. 2006;113(1):30–7. https://doi.org/10.1161/CIRCULATIONAHA.105. 580696.

39. Polonsky TS, McClelland RL, Jorgensen NW, Bild DE, Burke GL, Guerci AD, et al. Coronary artery calcium score and risk classification for coronary heart disease prediction. JAMA. 2010;303(16):1610–6. https://doi.org/10.1001/jama.2010.461.

40. Erbel R, Mohlenkamp S, Moebus S, Schmermund A, Lehmann N, Stang A, et al. Coronary risk stratification, discrimination, and reclassification improvement based on quantification

of subclinical coronary atherosclerosis: the Heinz Nixdorf Recall study. J Am Coll Cardiol. 2010;56(17):1397–406. https://doi.org/10.1016/j.jacc.2010.06.030.

41. Mohlenkamp S, Lehmann N, Moebus S, Schmermund A, Dragano N, Stang A, et al. Quantification of coronary atherosclerosis and inflammation to predict coronary events and all-cause mortality. J Am Coll Cardiol. 2011;57(13):1455–64. https://doi.org/10.1016/j.jacc.2010.10.043.

42. Elias-Smale SE, Proenca RV, Koller MT, Kavousi M, van Rooij FJ, Hunink MG, et al. Coronary calcium score improves classification of coronary heart disease risk in the elderly: the Rotterdam study. J Am Coll Cardiol. 2010;56(17):1407–14. https://doi.org/10.1016/j.jacc.2010.06.029.

43. Kavousi M, Desai CS, Ayers C, Blumenthal RS, Budoff MJ, Mahabadi AA, et al. Prevalence and prognostic implications of coronary artery calcification in low-risk women: a meta-analysis. JAMA. 2016;316(20):2126–34. https://doi.org/10.1001/jama.2016.17020.

44. Yano Y, O'Donnell CJ, Kuller L, Kavousi M, Erbel R, Ning H, et al. Association of coronary artery calcium score vs age with cardiovascular risk in older adults: an analysis of pooled population-based studies. JAMA Cardiol. 2017;2(9):986–94. https://doi.org/10.1001/jamacardio.2017.2498.

45. Nasir K, Bittencourt MS, Blaha MJ, Blankstein R, Agatson AS, Rivera JJ, et al. Implications of coronary artery calcium testing among statin candidates according to American college of cardiology/American heart association cholesterol management guidelines: MESA (Multi-Ethnic Study of Atherosclerosis). J Am Coll Cardiol. 2015;66(15):1657–68. https://doi.org/10.1016/j.jacc.2015.07.066.

46. Kianoush S, Mirbolouk M, Makam RC, Nasir K, Blaha MJ. Coronary artery calcium scoring in current clinical practice: how to define its value? Curr Treat Options Cardiovasc Med. 2017;19(11):85. https://doi.org/10.1007/s11936-017-0582-y.

47. Blaha MJ, Cainzos-Achirica M, Greenland P, McEvoy JW, Blankstein R, Budoff MJ, et al. Role of coronary artery calcium score of zero and other negative risk markers for cardiovascular disease: the Multi-Ethnic Study of Atherosclerosis (MESA). Circulation. 2016;133(9):849–58. https://doi.org/10.1161/CIRCULATIONAHA.115.018524.

48. Yeboah J, Polonsky TS, Young R, McClelland RL, Delaney JC, Dawood F, et al. Utility of nontraditional risk markers in individuals ineligible for statin therapy according to the 2013 American college of cardiology/American heart association cholesterol guidelines. Circulation. 2015;132(10):916–22. https://doi.org/10.1161/CIRCULATIONAHA.115.016846.

49. Yeboah J, McClelland RL, Polonsky TS, Burke GL, Sibley CT, O'Leary D, et al. Comparison of novel risk markers for improvement in cardiovascular risk assessment in intermediate-risk individuals. JAMA. 2012;308(8):788–95. https://doi.org/10.1001/jama.2012.9624.

50. Johnson JE, Gulanick M, Penckofer S, Kouba J. Does knowledge of coronary artery calcium affect cardiovascular risk perception, likelihood of taking action, and health-promoting behavior change? J Cardiovasc Nurs. 2015;30(1):15–25. https://doi.org/10.1097/JCN.0000000000000103.

51. Silverman MG, Blaha MJ, Krumholz HM, Budoff MJ, Blankstein R, Sibley CT, et al. Impact of coronary artery calcium on coronary heart disease events in individuals at the extremes of traditional risk factor burden: the multi-ethnic study of atherosclerosis. Eur Heart J. 2014;35(33):2232–41. https://doi.org/10.1093/eurheartj/eht508.

52. Blaha M, Budoff MJ, Shaw LJ, Khosa F, Rumberger JA, Berman D, et al. Absence of coronary artery calcification and all-cause mortality. JACC Cardiovasc Imaging. 2009;2(6):692–700. https://doi.org/10.1016/j.jcmg.2009.03.009.

53. Valenti V, B OH, Heo R, Cho I, Schulman-Marcus J, Gransar H, et al. A 15-Year Warranty Period for Asymptomatic Individuals Without Coronary Artery Calcium: A Prospective Follow-Up of 9,715 Individuals. JACC Cardiovasc Imaging. 2015;8(8):900–9. doi: https://doi.org/10.1016/j.jcmg.2015.01.025.

54. Valenti V, Hartaigh BO, Cho I, Schulman-Marcus J, Gransar H, Heo R, et al. Absence of coronary artery calcium identifies asymptomatic diabetic individuals at low near-term but not long-term risk of mortality: a 15-year follow-up study of 9715 patients. Circ Cardiovasc Imaging. 2016;9(2). https://doi.org/10.1161/CIRCIMAGING.115.003528.

55. Dzaye O, Dardari ZA, Cainzos-Achirica M, Blankstein R, Szklo M, Budoff MJ, et al. Incidence of new coronary calcification: time to conversion from CAC = 0. J Am Coll Cardiol. 2020;75(13):1610–3. https://doi.org/10.1016/j.jacc.2020.01.047.

56. Dzaye O, Dardari ZA, Cainzos-Achirica M, Blankstein R, Agatston AS, Duebgen M, et al. Warranty period of a calcium score of zero: comprehensive analysis from the multiethnic study of atherosclerosis. JACC Cardiovasc Imaging. 2020. https://doi.org/10.1016/j.jcmg.2020.06.048.

57. Desai CS, Ning H, Kang J, Folsom AR, Polak JF, Sibley CT, et al. Competing cardiovascular outcomes associated with subclinical atherosclerosis (from the Multi-Ethnic Study of Atherosclerosis). Am J Cardiol. 2013;111(11):1541–6. https://doi.org/10.1016/j.amjcard.2013.02.003.

58. Handy CE, Desai CS, Dardari ZA, Al-Mallah MH, Miedema MD, Ouyang P, et al. The association of coronary artery calcium with noncardiovascular disease: the multi-ethnic study of atherosclerosis. JACC Cardiovasc Imaging. 2016;9(5):568–76. https://doi.org/10.1016/j.jcmg.2015.09.020.

59. McClelland RL, Jorgensen NW, Budoff M, Blaha MJ, Post WS, Kronmal RA, et al. 10-year coronary heart disease risk prediction using coronary artery calcium and traditional risk factors: derivation in the MESA (Multi-Ethnic Study of Atherosclerosis) With Validation in the HNR (Heinz Nixdorf Recall) study and the DHS (Dallas Heart Study). J Am Coll Cardiol. 2015;66(15):1643–53. https://doi.org/10.1016/j.jacc.2015.08.035.

60. Eckert J, Schmidt M, Magedanz A, Voigtlander T, Schmermund A. Coronary CT angiography in managing atherosclerosis. Int J Mol Sci. 2015;16(2):3740–56. https://doi.org/10.3390/ijms16023740.

61. Kim KJ, Choi SI, Lee MS, Kim JA, Chun EJ, Jeon CH. The prevalence and characteristics of coronary atherosclerosis in asymptomatic subjects classified as low risk based on traditional risk stratification algorithm: assessment with coronary CT angiography. Heart. 2013;99(15):1113–7. https://doi.org/10.1136/heartjnl-2013-303631.

62. Leber AW, Knez A, White CW, Becker A, von Ziegler F, Muehling O, et al. Composition of coronary atherosclerotic plaques in patients with acute myocardial infarction and stable angina pectoris determined by contrast-enhanced multislice computed tomography. Am J Cardiol. 2003;91(6):714–8. https://doi.org/10.1016/s0002-9149(02)03411-2.

63. Hulten E, Bittencourt MS, Ghoshhajra B, O'Leary D, Christman MP, Blaha MJ, et al. Incremental prognostic value of coronary artery calcium score versus CT angiography among symptomatic patients without known coronary artery disease. Atherosclerosis. 2014;233(1):190–5. https://doi.org/10.1016/j.atherosclerosis.2013.12.029.

64. Sarwar A, Shaw LJ, Shapiro MD, Blankstein R, Hoffmann U, Cury RC, et al. Diagnostic and prognostic value of absence of coronary artery calcification. JACC Cardiovasc Imaging. 2009;2(6):675–88. https://doi.org/10.1016/j.jcmg.2008.12.031.

65. Villines TC, Hulten EA, Shaw LJ, Goyal M, Dunning A, Achenbach S, et al. Prevalence and severity of coronary artery disease and adverse events among symptomatic patients with coronary artery calcification scores of zero undergoing coronary computed tomography angiography: results from the CONFIRM (Coronary CT Angiography Evaluation for Clinical Outcomes: An International Multicenter) registry. J Am Coll Cardiol. 2011;58(24):2533–40. https://doi.org/10.1016/j.jacc.2011.10.851.

66. Motoyama S, Sarai M, Harigaya H, Anno H, Inoue K, Hara T, et al. Computed tomographic angiography characteristics of atherosclerotic plaques subsequently resulting in acute coronary syndrome. J Am Coll Cardiol. 2009;54(1):49–57. https://doi.org/10.1016/j.jacc.2009.02.068.

67. Hemal K, Pagidipati NJ, Coles A, Dolor RJ, Mark DB, Pellikka PA, et al. Sex differences in demographics, risk factors, presentation, and noninvasive testing in stable outpatients with

suspected coronary artery disease: insights from the PROMISE Trial. JACC Cardiovasc Imaging. 2016;9(4):337–46. https://doi.org/10.1016/j.jcmg.2016.02.001.

68. Ferencik M, Schlett CL, Ghoshhajra BB, Kriegel MF, Joshi SB, Maurovich-Horvat P, et al. A computed tomography-based coronary lesion score to predict acute coronary syndrome among patients with acute chest pain and significant coronary stenosis on coronary computed tomographic angiogram. Am J Cardiol. 2012;110(2):183–9. https://doi.org/10.1016/j.amjcard.2012.02.066.

69. Leipsic J, Abbara S, Achenbach S, Cury R, Earls JP, Mancini GJ, et al. SCCT guidelines for the interpretation and reporting of coronary CT angiography: a report of the society of cardiovascular computed tomography guidelines committee. J Cardiovasc Comput Tomogr. 2014;8(5):342–58. https://doi.org/10.1016/j.jcct.2014.07.003.

70. Hadamitzky M, Achenbach S, Al-Mallah M, Berman D, Budoff M, Cademartiri F, et al. Optimized prognostic score for coronary computed tomographic angiography: results from the CONFIRM registry (COronary CT Angiography EvaluatioN For Clinical Outcomes: An InteRnational Multicenter Registry). J Am Coll Cardiol. 2013;62(5):468–76. https://doi.org/10.1016/j.jacc.2013.04.064.

71. Mortensen MB, Steffensen FH, Botker HE, Jensen JM, Ronnow Sand NP, Kragholm KH, et al. CAD severity on cardiac CTA identifies patients with most benefit of treating LDL-cholesterol to ACC/AHA and ESC/EAS targets. JACC Cardiovasc Imaging. 2020;13 (9):1961–72. https://doi.org/10.1016/j.jcmg.2020.03.017.

72. Douglas PS, Hoffmann U, Patel MR, Mark DB, Al-Khalidi HR, Cavanaugh B, et al. Outcomes of anatomical versus functional testing for coronary artery disease. N Engl J Med. 2015;372(14):1291–300. https://doi.org/10.1056/NEJMoa1415516.

73. Adamson PD, Newby DE. The SCOT-HEART Trial. What we observed and what we learned. J Cardiovasc Comput Tomogr. 2019;13(3):54–8. doi: https://doi.org/10.1016/j.jcct.2019.01.006.

74. Lubbers M, Dedic A, Coenen A, Galema T, Akkerhuis J, Bruning T, et al. Calcium imaging and selective computed tomography angiography in comparison to functional testing for suspected coronary artery disease: the multicentre, randomized CRESCENT trial. Eur Heart J. 2016;37(15):1232–43. https://doi.org/10.1093/eurheartj/ehv700.

75. Plank F, Friedrich G, Dichtl W, Klauser A, Jaschke W, Franz WM, et al. The diagnostic and prognostic value of coronary CT angiography in asymptomatic high-risk patients: a cohort study. Open Heart. 2014;1(1). https://doi.org/10.1136/openhrt-2014-000096.

76. Muhlestein JB, Lappe DL, Lima JA, Rosen BD, May HT, Knight S, et al. Effect of screening for coronary artery disease using CT angiography on mortality and cardiac events in high-risk patients with diabetes: the FACTOR-64 randomized clinical trial. JAMA. 2014;312(21):2234–43. https://doi.org/10.1001/jama.2014.15825.

77. Cho I, Chang HJ, Sung JM, Pencina MJ, Lin FY, Dunning AM, et al. Coronary computed tomographic angiography and risk of all-cause mortality and nonfatal myocardial infarction in subjects without chest pain syndrome from the CONFIRM registry (coronary CT angiography evaluation for clinical outcomes: an international multicenter registry). Circulation. 2012;126(3):304–13. https://doi.org/10.1161/CIRCULATIONAHA.111.081380.

78. Zhao X, Zhao Q, Chu B, Yang Y, Li F, Zhou XH, et al. Prevalence of compositional features in subclinical carotid atherosclerosis determined by high-resolution magnetic resonance imaging in chinese patients with coronary artery disease. Stroke. 2010;41(6):1157–62. https://doi.org/10.1161/STROKEAHA.110.580027.

79. Kablak-Ziembicka A, Tracz W, Przewlocki T, Pieniazek P, Sokolowski A, Konieczynska M. Association of increased carotid intima-media thickness with the extent of coronary artery disease. Heart. 2004;90(11):1286–90. https://doi.org/10.1136/hrt.2003.025080.

80. Lekakis JP, Papamichael CM, Cimponeriu AT, Stamatelopoulos KS, Papaioannou TG, Kanakakis J, et al. Atherosclerotic changes of extracoronary arteries are associated with the extent of coronary atherosclerosis. Am J Cardiol. 2000;85(8):949–52. https://doi.org/10.1016/s0002-9149(99)00907-8.

                                                                O. Dzaye et al.

81. Nagai Y, Metter EJ, Earley CJ, Kemper MK, Becker LC, Lakatta EG, et al. Increased carotid artery intimal-medial thickness in asymptomatic older subjects with exercise-induced myocardial ischemia. Circulation. 1998;98(15):1504–9. https://doi.org/10.1161/01.cir.98.15.1504.

82. Spence JD. Technology Insight: ultrasound measurement of carotid plaque–patient management, genetic research, and therapy evaluation. Nat Clin Pract Neurol. 2006;2(11):611–9. https://doi.org/10.1038/ncpneuro0324.

83. Spence JD, Hegele RA. Noninvasive phenotypes of atherosclerosis: similar windows but different views. Stroke. 2004;35(3):649–53. https://doi.org/10.1161/01.STR.0000116103.19029.DB.

84. Stein JH, Korcarz CE, Hurst RT, Lonn E, Kendall CB, Mohler ER, et al. Use of carotid ultrasound to identify subclinical vascular disease and evaluate cardiovascular disease risk: a consensus statement from the American society of echocardiography carotid intima-media Thickness task force. endorsed by the society for vascular medicine. J Am Soc Echocardiogr. 2008;21(2):93–111; quiz 89–90. doi: https://doi.org/10.1016/j.echo.2007.11.011.

85. Inaba Y, Chen JA, Bergmann SR. Carotid plaque, compared with carotid intima-media thickness, more accurately predicts coronary artery disease events: a meta-analysis. Atherosclerosis. 2012;220(1):128–33. https://doi.org/10.1016/j.atherosclerosis.2011.06.044.

86. Den Ruijter HM, Peters SA, Anderson TJ, Britton AR, Dekker JM, Eijkemans MJ, et al. Common carotid intima-media thickness measurements in cardiovascular risk prediction: a meta-analysis. JAMA. 2012;308(8):796–803. https://doi.org/10.1001/jama.2012.9630.

87. Folsom AR, Kronmal RA, Detrano RC, O'Leary DH, Bild DE, Bluemke DA, et al. Coronary artery calcification compared with carotid intima-media thickness in the prediction of cardiovascular disease incidence: the Multi-Ethnic Study of Atherosclerosis (MESA). Arch Intern Med. 2008;168(12):1333–9. https://doi.org/10.1001/archinte.168.12.1333.

88. Bots ML, Groenewegen KA, Anderson TJ, Britton AR, Dekker JM, Engstrom G, et al. Common carotid intima-media thickness measurements do not improve cardiovascular risk prediction in individuals with elevated blood pressure: the USE-IMT collaboration. Hypertension. 2014;63(6):1173–81. https://doi.org/10.1161/HYPERTENSIONAHA.113.02683.

89. Simon A, Megnien JL, Chironi G. The value of carotid intima-media thickness for predicting cardiovascular risk. Arterioscler Thromb Vasc Biol. 2010;30(2):182–5. https://doi.org/10.1161/ATVBAHA.109.196980.

90. Authors/Task Force M, Piepoli MF, Hoes AW, Agewall S, Albus C, Brotons C, et al. 2016 European guidelines on cardiovascular disease prevention in clinical practice: the sixth joint task force of the European society of cardiology and other societies on cardiovascular disease prevention in clinical practice (constituted by representatives of 10 societies and by invited experts) developed with the special contribution of the European Association for Cardiovascular Prevention & Rehabilitation (EACPR). Atherosclerosis. 2016;252:207–74. doi: https://doi.org/10.1016/j.atherosclerosis.2016.05.037.

91. Geerts CC, Bots ML, van der Ent CK, Grobbee DE, Uiterwaal CS. Parental smoking and vascular damage in their 5-year-old children. Pediatrics. 2012;129(1):45–54. https://doi.org/10.1542/peds.2011-0249.

92. Evelein AM, Geerts CC, Bots ML, van der Ent CK, Grobbee DE, Uiterwaal CS. Parental blood pressure is related to vascular properties of their 5-year-old offspring. Am J Hypertens. 2012;25(8):907–13. https://doi.org/10.1038/ajh.2012.66.

93. Tison GH, Guo M, Blaha MJ, McClelland RL, Allison MA, Szklo M, et al. Multisite extracoronary calcification indicates increased risk of coronary heart disease and all-cause mortality: the multi-ethnic study of atherosclerosis. J Cardiovasc Comput Tomogr. 2015;9(5):406–14. https://doi.org/10.1016/j.jcct.2015.03.012.

94. Gondrie MJ, van der Graaf Y, Jacobs PC, Oen AL, Mali WP, Group PS. The association of incidentally detected heart valve calcification with future cardiovascular events. Eur Radiol. 2011;21(5):963–73. doi: https://doi.org/10.1007/s00330-010-1995-0.

95. Iribarren C, Sidney S, Sternfeld B, Browner WS. Calcification of the aortic arch: risk factors and association with coronary heart disease, stroke, and peripheral vascular disease. JAMA. 2000;283(21):2810–5. https://doi.org/10.1001/jama.283.21.2810.

96. Barasch E, Gottdiener JS, Marino Larsen EK, Chaves PH, Newman AB. Cardiovascular morbidity and mortality in community-dwelling elderly individuals with calcification of the fibrous skeleton of the base of the heart and aortosclerosis (The Cardiovascular Health Study). Am J Cardiol. 2006;97(9):1281–6. https://doi.org/10.1016/j.amjcard.2005.11.065.

97. Makris GC, Teng Z, Patterson AJ, Lin JM, Young V, Graves MJ, et al. Advances in MRI for the evaluation of carotid atherosclerosis. Br J Radiol. 2015;88(1052):20140282. https://doi.org/10.1259/bjr.20140282.

98. Naghavi M, Libby P, Falk E, Casscells SW, Litovsky S, Rumberger J, et al. From vulnerable plaque to vulnerable patient: a call for new definitions and risk assessment strategies: Part II. Circulation. 2003;108(15):1772–8. https://doi.org/10.1161/01.CIR.0000087481.55887.C9.

99. Spagnoli LG, Mauriello A, Sangiorgi G, Fratoni S, Bonanno E, Schwartz RS, et al. Extracranial thrombotically active carotid plaque as a risk factor for ischemic stroke. JAMA. 2004;292(15):1845–52. https://doi.org/10.1001/jama.292.15.1845.

100. Saam T, Hetterich H, Hoffmann V, Yuan C, Dichgans M, Poppert H, et al. Meta-analysis and systematic review of the predictive value of carotid plaque hemorrhage on cerebrovascular events by magnetic resonance imaging. J Am Coll Cardiol. 2013;62(12):1081–91. https://doi.org/10.1016/j.jacc.2013.06.015.

101. Daghem M, Bing R, Fayad ZA, Dweck MR. Noninvasive imaging to assess atherosclerotic plaque composition and disease activity: coronary and carotid applications. JACC Cardiovasc Imaging. 2020;13(4):1055–68. https://doi.org/10.1016/j.jcmg.2019.03.033.

102. Zavodni AE, Wasserman BA, McClelland RL, Gomes AS, Folsom AR, Polak JF, et al. Carotid artery plaque morphology and composition in relation to incident cardiovascular events: the Multi-Ethnic Study of Atherosclerosis (MESA). Radiology. 2014;271(2):381–9. https://doi.org/10.1148/radiol.14131020.

103. Dweck MR, Chow MW, Joshi NV, Williams MC, Jones C, Fletcher AM, et al. Coronary arterial 18F-sodium fluoride uptake: a novel marker of plaque biology. J Am Coll Cardiol. 2012;59(17):1539–48. https://doi.org/10.1016/j.jacc.2011.12.037.

104. Tarkin JM, Joshi FR, Evans NR, Chowdhury MM, Figg NL, Shah AV, et al. Detection of atherosclerotic inflammation by (68)Ga-DOTATATE PET compared to [(18)F]FDG PET Imaging. J Am Coll Cardiol. 2017;69(14):1774–91. https://doi.org/10.1016/j.jacc.2017.01.060.

105. Dorbala S, Di Carli MF, Beanlands RS, Merhige ME, Williams BA, Veledar E, et al. Prognostic value of stress myocardial perfusion positron emission tomography: results from a multicenter observational registry. J Am Coll Cardiol. 2013;61(2):176–84. https://doi.org/10.1016/j.jacc.2012.09.043.

106. Yoshinaga K, Chow BJ, Williams K, Chen L, deKemp RA, Garrard L, et al. What is the prognostic value of myocardial perfusion imaging using rubidium-82 positron emission tomography? J Am Coll Cardiol. 2006;48(5):1029–39. https://doi.org/10.1016/j.jacc.2006.06.025.

107. Young LH, Wackers FJ, Chyun DA, Davey JA, Barrett EJ, Taillefer R, et al. Cardiac outcomes after screening for asymptomatic coronary artery disease in patients with type 2 diabetes: the DIAD study: a randomized controlled trial. JAMA. 2009;301(15):1547–55. https://doi.org/10.1001/jama.2009.476.

108. Berman DS, Wong ND, Gransar H, Miranda-Peats R, Dahlbeck J, Hayes SW, et al. Relationship between stress-induced myocardial ischemia and atherosclerosis measured by coronary calcium tomography. J Am Coll Cardiol. 2004;44(4):923–30. https://doi.org/10.1016/j.jacc.2004.06.042.

109. Rozanski A, Berman DS. The synergistic use of coronary artery calcium imaging and noninvasive myocardial perfusion imaging for detecting subclinical atherosclerosis and myocardial ischemia. Curr Cardiol Rep. 2018;20(7):59. https://doi.org/10.1007/s11886-018-1001-z.

110. Schmermund A, Achenbach S, Budde T, Buziashvili Y, Forster A, Friedrich G, et al. Effect of intensive versus standard lipid-lowering treatment with atorvastatin on the progression of calcified coronary atherosclerosis over 12 months: a multicenter, randomized, double-blind trial. Circulation. 2006;113(3):427–37. https://doi.org/10.1161/CIRCULATIONAHA.105.568147.

111. Wong ND, Rozanski A, Gransar H, Miranda-Peats R, Kang X, Hayes S, et al. Metabolic syndrome and diabetes are associated with an increased likelihood of inducible myocardial ischemia among patients with subclinical atherosclerosis. Diabetes Care. 2005;28(6):1445–50. https://doi.org/10.2337/diacare.28.6.1445.

112. Sundstrom J, Lind L, Arnlov J, Zethelius B, Andren B, Lithell HO. Echocardiographic and electrocardiographic diagnoses of left ventricular hypertrophy predict mortality independently of each other in a population of elderly men. Circulation. 2001;103(19):2346–51. https://doi.org/10.1161/01.cir.103.19.2346.

113. Michos ED, Abraham TP. Echoing the appropriate use criteria: the role of echocardiography for cardiovascular risk assessment of the asymptomatic individual. JAMA Intern Med. 2013;173(17):1598–9. https://doi.org/10.1001/jamainternmed.2013.7029.

114. Maroules CD, Khera A, Ayers C, Goel A, Peshock RM, Abbara S, et al. Cardiovascular outcome associations among cardiovascular magnetic resonance measures of arterial stiffness: the Dallas heart study. J Cardiovasc Magn Reson. 2014;16:33. https://doi.org/10.1186/1532-429X-16-33.

115. Blaha MJ, Blumenthal RS, Budoff MJ, Nasir K. Understanding the utility of zero coronary calcium as a prognostic test: a Bayesian approach. Circ Cardiovasc Qual Outcomes. 2011;4(2):253–6. https://doi.org/10.1161/CIRCOUTCOMES.110.958496.

Digital Health

Francoise A. Marvel, Pauline P. Huynh, and Seth S. Martin

Introduction

As the digital ecosystem continues to grow in the United States (US), it is estimated that there will be over 50 billion internet-connected devices by 2020 with 91% of the US population owning smartphones by 2025 [1]. The traditional approach to cardiovascular disease (CVD) management is being disrupted by unprecedented levels of innovation focusing on enhanced systems of healthcare delivery, patient engagement, tracking, and virtual health coaching through state-of-the-art consumer-based technology called digital health interventions (DHIs). DHIs are defined by the US Food and Drug Administration (FDA) as any form of software or hardware used to improve the quality, access, efficacy, or efficiency of health care delivery [2]. The World Health Organization (WHO) Global Observatory for eHealth (GOe) uses a broader definition of mobile health (mHealth) as medical and public health practice supported by mobile devices [3]. The rapid evolution of health-related digital technologies has the potential to synergize with principles of precision medicine. This convergence of health technology and precision medicine is impacting healthcare delivery and may prove to be a cost-effective solution for cardiovascular disease detection, management, and health equity. This chapter discusses state-of-the-digital science for delivery of personalized care. Specifically the following topics are addressed: (1) consumer connected health and tracking, (2) digital health coaching, and (3) transformation of healthcare delivery.

F. A. Marvel · P. P. Huynh · S. S. Martin (✉)
Digital Health Innovation Laboratory, Ciccarone Center for the Prevention of Cardiovascular Disease, Division of Cardiology, Department of Medicine, Johns Hopkins University School of Medicine, Johns Hopkins Hospital, 600 N. Wolfe St., Carnegie 568, Baltimore, MD 21287, US
e-mail: smart100@jhmi.edu

© Springer Nature Switzerland AG 2021
S. S. Martin (ed.), *Precision Medicine in Cardiovascular Disease Prevention*, https://doi.org/10.1007/978-3-030-75055-8_5

Consumer Connected Health & Tracking

The economic success of the digital health technology market is emblematic of society's interest in consumer-empowered health transformation and disease prevention [4–6]. As technologies advance, consumers are able to access and track additional health metrics (heart rate, blood pressure, weight, oxygen saturation), biomarkers (blood glucose), physical activity (step count, frequency, duration, and type of exercise), and adherence to treatment goals (medication adherence, diet) [6, 7]. In 2017 alone, there existed over 350,000 mHealth apps spanning calorie count and exercise regimens, allowing for manual logging of diet and exercise [8]. Moreover, given increasing patient interest in sharing health data from smart devices with their clinicians, [9] the ability to access these ambulatory data could serve as a valuable asset in developing an individualized care plan. For example, longitudinal data collected from these devices will allow clinicians to titrate medication dosages based on a range of readings versus one set collected at time of office visit thereby increasing patient safety and improving outcomes [6]. Within cardiovascular medicine, there have been a multitude of studies evaluating the breadth and efficacy of these technologies, as detailed below and summarized in Fig. 1. Below, we highlight examples of major advances in innovation and clinical trials of these technologies.

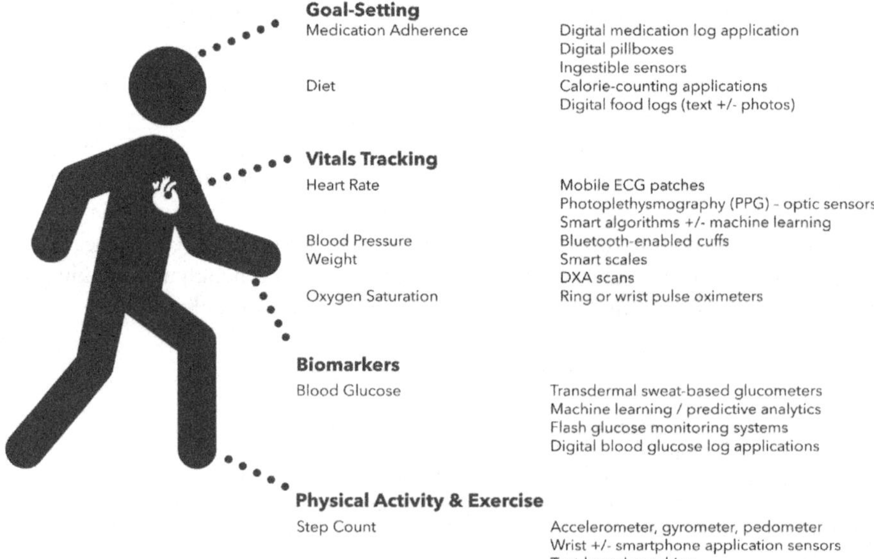

Fig. 1 Summary of consumer connected health tools and tracking technologies

Heart Rate Monitoring and Arrhythmia Detection

Since 2017, the FDA has cleared several digital health apps and devices targeting heart rhythm monitoring, bringing these technologies directly in the hands of consumers [10–16]. Many of these apps and devices utilize mobile external electrocardiograms (ECGs), [14] optic technology such as photoplethysmography (PPG) that detects pulsatile light changes in the vascular bed beneath the skin, [13] and smart algorithms to record heart rates and even alert users of irregular heart rhythms such as atrial fibrillation (AF). Other innovations have included a dermal self-applied ECG patch [4].

We can infer the popularity of these features among consumers given the rapid flux of releases and 510(K) applications [10–16]. For example, in 2018, the FDA approved an ECG app and irregular heart rhythm notification feature on the Apple Watch; this was followed by a series of approvals for the AliveCor KardiaMobile, marketed as "a personal EKG" for the detection of atrial fibrillation, bradycardia, and tachycardia [13, 14, 17]. It is therefore imperative that the information from these devices and applications are validated, given the clinical significance of heart rate data in diagnosing and managing cardiac arrhythmias. In their review, Al-Alusi et al. [18] describe 11 devices specifically targeting cardiac monitoring, noting the swaths of studies supporting the validity of the Apple Watch and AliveCor Kardia devices to detect AF. Beyond accurate detection, however, the authors highlight the need for studies evaluating the use of these wearables on patient outcomes as well as the need for collaboration between clinicians and manufacturers for clinical integration [19–21]. In response to the call for integration of health technology into clinical workflow, innovative teams are developing clinical decision support tools based on machine learning algorithms from user-generated data [7, 22].

Blood Pressure Tracking

In addition to heart rate monitoring, the advancement of wearables also allows for remote blood pressure (BP) tracking through wireless Bluetooth-enabled cuffs. BP control is a major risk factor for cardiovascular health and unfortunately nearly half (46%) of the adult US population have hypertension according to the most recent AHA/ACC guidelines [23]. Effective BP management strategies have generally integrated patient education, medication reminders, and behavioral modification [7, 24]. Although patients are encouraged to measure and record their BP at home, multiple studies have found these logs to substantially under-report BP when compared to measurements done in a clinical setting, [25] and that self-tracking alone is insufficient without education or medical decision-making in response to those measurements [26, 27]. Initial efforts to leverage telemedicine in BP management have included reminder systems and coaching programs; however, these efforts were limited by a commitment on behalf of the patient to manually measure their BP and transmit their recorded measurements to clinic via fax, email, or paper logs [28–30].

More recent innovations have included automated BP measurements through a Bluetooth-enabled cuff, which could be paired with a smartphone application to store measurements [4, 31]. Like with HR data, these devices have the potential to generate enormous amounts of BP data that could provide actionable insights and facilitate personalized medical decision-making, including systematic medication titration, if properly integrated in clinical workflow. In their randomized clinical trial, Rifkin et al. [30] demonstrated the feasibility of a home-based Bluetooth-enabled BP monitoring for older patients through the use of wirelessly transmitted BP readings to their care team. Patients who were randomized into the digital intervention arm transmitted a median of 29 BP readings to their clinician per month, allowing for interval titration of their medication regimen by their care team and achieving overall better BP control over the course of 6 months. This study highlights how digital technology could synergize with precision medicine among patients with cardiovascular disease, including hypertension, while demonstrating patients' willingness to utilize these technologies over the long term.

Weight Tracking and Management

The rising prevalence of obesity has reached epidemic levels, affecting over 90 million people in the United States or 1 in 3 Americans [32]. In addition to higher rates of morbidity and mortality, obesity has been consistently associated with cardiovascular disease [33]. Furthermore, these health risks could be significantly mitigated with as little as a 5–10% weight loss [34, 35]. Unfortunately, despite numerous weight loss interventions spanning lifestyle modification, pharmacology, and surgery, long-term efficacy remains elusive [36, 37]. The heterogeneity of responses has been attributed to the multifactorial mechanism of obesity, involving the interplay of genetic and environmental factors. As a result, attention has turned to precision medicine as a potential solution to account for these variables and promote sustainable weight management [38].

Interestingly, while precision medicine is conventionally known to consider genetic differences in formulating interventions, discussions of its application for weight loss extended beyond pharmacological efficacy into strategies optimizing long-term patient adherence and sustainable lifestyle modification [38, 39]. These strategies may include the frequency of communication between the patient and healthcare team, cost of intervention (e.g. medication, gym membership, level of supervision), or intervention intensity. Moreover, Severin et al. [38] notes that technological advances may be a cost-effective solution to address potential barriers.

Outside of targeted weight loss programs, there is a growing desire among the public to know more about their weight, body compositions, and ways to optimize their fitness goals. This is evidenced by the rising market for DXA scans as promoted on social media platforms as a way to personalize weight loss goals. Consumer connected health technologies have capitalized on this desire, empowering users to track and log their weight, with some even breaking the weight down into muscle mass, water, and fat. However, the validity of these consumer weight analytics remains unknown, [40] highlighting a need for further research.

Medication Adherence Support and Tracking

For individuals with CVD and related risk factors, medical therapy is a mainstay of management along with lifestyle modification. Unfortunately, medication adherence remains a challenge for a majority of patients [41] and poses a substantial economic burden, translating into over $5 billion in preventable costs annually and poor outcomes [42]. Conventional methods of evaluating adherence are limited by their subjective (e.g. recall bias), time-consuming (e.g. manual pill count), and cost (e.g. obtaining serum levels) [43]. Advances of digital technologies and connected health devices may provide a cost-effective solution to optimize medication adherence through patient empowerment, education, and communication.

Multiple interventions targeting medication adherence have been developed including remote medication delivery, scheduled text message or push notification reminders to take medication, and even medication intake surveillance. The Corrie Health Digital Platform, as an example, features a medication log with relevant information about each medication, a notification system of when to take medications, and a visual summarizing adherence information [44]. Other examples have included digital pillboxes and "digitized medicine" with ingestible sensors verifying medication adherence with information synced to a provider portal [45, 46]. Although aimed to improve adherence, the invasive nature of digital pills has sparked ethical debate on patient autonomy [47]. Furthermore, while a systematic review by Conway & Kelechi [43] found some of these strategies to increase adherence in the short-term, long-term adherence to therapy remains unknown as most studies have a maximum follow-up of only 6 months. As these technologies continue to develop, it is imperative that industry leaders collaborate with clinicians to ensure long-term efficacy and preserve the patient-clinician relationship.

Physical Activity and Exercise Tracking

There exists a plethora of connected health technologies—from pedometers to smartwatches to wrist step sensors to smartphone applications—aimed at promoting and tracking physical activity and exercise. These technologies provide objective data on intensity and duration of activity, as well as feedback on user's progress toward their daily fitness goals. While these digital solutions may involve personalized coaching and automated activity tracking described in further detail later in this chapter, there remains a need to promote actionable insights for behavior change. Moreover, although these technologies have been associated with short-term increases in activity and even weight reduction, [48–50] the long-term efficacy on outcomes remain equivocal [51].

Diet and Nutrition Tracking

Within the digital health sphere, diet self-tracking has been primarily used within the health prevention and personal fitness space, as demonstrated by the growing number of food diary and calorie-counting applications [52]. This highlights the common theme of digital consumers attempting to leverage digital tools and optimize their own health and wellness; indeed, several diet-related mobile applications offer nutrition recommendations based on user-entered biometric data (e.g. height, weight, activity level) and fitness goals (e.g. weight loss, gain muscle mass). Users of these applications can track their own dietary intake, leveraging extensive food databases via barcode scans on their smartphones or manually enter nutrition information. Other innovative approaches allow users to take photos of each food or meal, logging them into a digital diary [53].

Given AHA/ACC recommended cardiac diets (i.e. DASH, sodium-restriction) in cardiovascular disease prevention and management, research efforts have recently focused on the accuracy of the data in these connected health technologies and their efficacy, especially in patients with chronic disease. In their review of the 7 most popular diet-tracking mobile applications, Ferrara et al. [54] found that although most diet-tracking applications scored well in terms of usability and goal-oriented behavior change there was inconsistency in the information provided. Specifically, they found variability in nutrient estimates when compared to those provided by the US Department of Agriculture as well as differences between the iOS and Android versions of the same applications. Based on this summary, further investigations on the validity of nutrition facts provided by consumer diet-tracking tools is needed.

Digital Biomarker Tracking

The rapid digital and technology advances have allowed consumers access to their own information, including physiological measures. Digital biomarkers are consumer-generated physiological and behavioral measures collected through connected digital tools. Two such examples are continuous transdermal glucose readings for patients with diabetes and remote monitoring of pulmonary artery pressure for patients with congestive heart failure.

It has been well-established that diabetes mellitus is a major risk factor for cardiovascular diseases, [55, 56] with a seminal study describing its risk of as equivalent to a non-diabetic with a history of myocardial infarction [57–59]. However, while routine measurement of one's blood glucose, often through finger-prick blood samples using a lancet, is part of standard of care to ensure adequate glucose control, the discomfort with glucose testing and cost of testing supplies has highlighted a need to develop accurate non-invasive methods to measure glucose concentrations [60]. Digital health technology advancements may be uniquely apt at addressing the need for painless monitoring, as demonstrated by the recent development of mobile glucometers and transdermal sensors. Additionally, the ability to continuous monitor blood glucose vs. discrete glucose monitoring may present an opportunity for further personalizing and optimizing glucose management for a patient.

In 2018, Segman [61] released a methods paper describing the technology behind the Cogna TensorTip Combo Glucometer, a device containing invasive and non-invasive components via optic technology and mathematical modeling for glucose monitoring. Another unobtrusive method involved transdermal sweat-based glucose monitoring through disposable sensor patches, correcting for skin temperature and humidity [62]. Recently, there have also been attempts to leverage machine learning in personalized blood glucose prediction, although challenges remain in developing universal algorithms to predict hyper- and hypo-glycemic events [63]. Lastly, while technically invasive, a third area of research focuses on flash glucose monitoring systems, which utilize a subcutaneous sensor to take scheduled measurements of the interstitial fluid glucose concentration as frequently as every minute and can be monitored in real time [64]. One notable example of a flash glucose monitoring system is the Freestyle Libre system, which has been associated with high user satisfaction, although data on long-term clinical and quality of life outcomes are lacking [65].

Another use case of a hybrid approach of remote physiologic monitoring combined with digital health is an implantable continuous monitor of pulmonary arterial pressure for early identification of volume overload in heart failure patients [66]. With the advent of consumer connected health trackers and patient portals, both patients and clinicians can now have access to this clinical information, as demonstrated by Abbott's CardioMEMS HF System, which comprises of an implantable remote monitor measuring pulmonary arterial pressure, a mobile application for the patient, and a clinician portal through a collaboration with the Merlin system [67]. The robust network demonstrated by this system highlights how the ability to proactively monitor biomarkers and adjust for individual patient thresholds could transform the healthcare system, reducing hospitalizations as much as 33–50% [66].

Digital Health Coaching

Overview of Digital Health Coaching

The approach to designing and developing mHealth coaching tools is based on the combination of clinical expertise and widely accepted theories promoting health behavior change. The two most common theories for behavioral change in mHealth are the Health Belief Model (HBM) and social cognitive theory [68]. The HBM theorizes that people's beliefs about whether they are at risk for a health problem, and their perceived benefits of taking action, influence readiness to change [69]. The HBM has most frequently been applied for prevention-related, asymptomatic conditions such as CVD [70, 71]. The social cognitive theory synthesizes concepts from cognitive, behavioristic, and emotional models of behavior change and can be applied to interventions for disease prevention and management [72]. Both theoretical approaches have overlapping constructs that, when included in behavior change interventions, have been associated with better outcomes [73–77]. Behavior change strategies based on these theories, such as education, self-monitoring, goal-setting, feedback, and prompts, are particularly useful components of mHealth interventions. A review of 13 lifestyle activity monitors show that the majority employ a variety of behavior change techniques, including self monitoring feedback, goal setting, behavioral cues, and rewards for past success [78].

Digital health coaching begins with the patient embedded in a health ecosystem (cardiovascular disease, risk behaviors, social determinants of health, and genetics) and utilizing health technology as self-monitoring health improvement strategy. The next level of coaching occurs when health data is captured and transmitted to the patient's digital health care network to inform coaching and management decisions. The following figure illustrates the mechanism of action and workflow of digital health coaching to individualize care (Fig. 2).

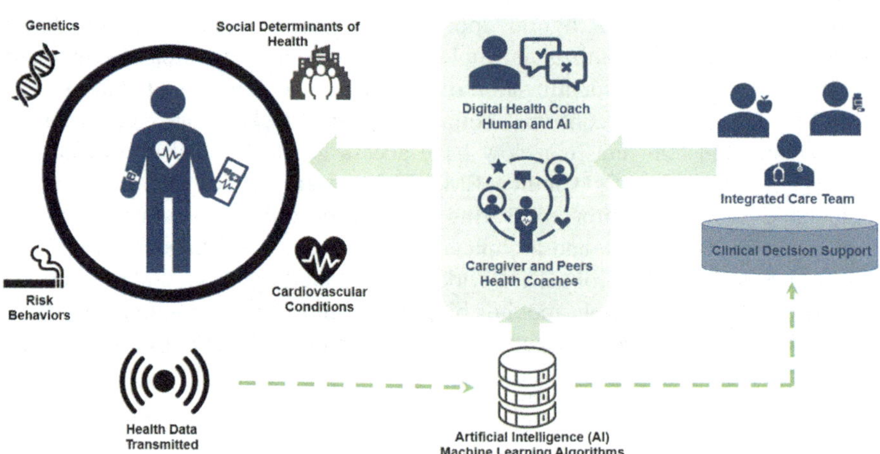

Fig. 2 Digital health coaching mechanism of action

Exercise Health Coaching

A key example of mHealth exercise health coaching is the mActive randomized clinical trial in which Martin et al. evaluated the ability of an automated and personalized text messaging system to increase physical activity [48]. The text messages were customized to an individual's schedule and real-time level of physical activity, among other personal factors such as name and favorite athlete (e.g., "Jon, you are on track to have a VERY ACTIVE day! Outstanding! We might as well call you Lebron James!"). 48 patients from the Johns Hopkins Ciccarone Center for the Prevention of Heart Disease participated, including some with cardiovascular disease risk factors such as diabetes and some with known coronary heart disease, thus targeting both primary and secondary prevention. Using a sequential randomization design, Martin et al. evaluated two core interventions: activity tracking and text messaging [48]. Activity outcomes were similar in patients who could access the activity tracker data in real-time (unblinded) as compared with those who could not (blinded to real-time activity data but wore the same tracker). There was a 25% increase in physical activity (~ 1 mile per day increase) when patients received automated coaching via personalized text messages, thereby supporting the need for such motivational drivers in addition to simple self-monitoring with devices. A systematic review of 11 articles similarly showed promise for electronic activity systems (wearables) to increase physical activity and manage weight [79].

Smoking Cessation Coaching

Smoking has long been recognized as a major risk factor for CVD and a leading preventable cause of death [7]. Moreover, successful attempts at smoking cessation have conventionally applied behavior change techniques [80]. Digital devices and mobile technologies have allowed for the scaling of these behavioral intervention at the convenience of device ownership, thereby having the potential to reach an impact at the population level. This has been noted by the immense number of text message-based cessation programs, including the American Cancer Society's Text2Quit and National Cancer Institute's SmokeFreeTXT programs [7, 81–84]. These programs have been shown to successfully leverage remote support, education counseling, and scheduled messages in order to promote and maintain smoking cessation [81, 84, 85]. Moreover, there is potential to promote a "precision" framework through personalized messaging, timed to situational urges such as around one's scheduled work breaks—when the risks of relapse are high—as described in the "just-in-time" adaptive interventions [86]. These efforts may be further augmented when deployed in combination with live support through telephone counseling [87].

Blood Pressure Control Coaching

According to recent American Heart Association guidelines, 103 million U.S. adults (about 46%) have hypertension, costing the healthcare system about $48.9 billion annually. In 2005, hypertension was responsible for 45% of all cardiovascular deaths, making it the single largest cardiovascular risk factor [88]. As discussed in this chapter, there remains ample opportunity to leverage digital health technologies within a precision medicine framework to facilitate personalized care. One such avenue is through mHealth coaching, as demonstrated in remote blood pressure management. A meta-analysis showed that self-monitoring of blood pressure alone improves hypertension control and the effect is greater for programs combining self-monitoring with additional support [89]. Virtual strategies including low-cost wireless monitoring is another example of traditional office-based appointments being transitioned to virtual visits. As demonstrated by Rifkin et al., remote wireless transmission of BP measurements from a Bluetooth-enabled cuff allowed for more frequent medication titrations, resulting in greater communication between the care team and patient as well as a trend toward improvements in BP control over usual care at 6 months [30]. A more recent retrospective study expanded on the potential utility of mHealth coaching in promoting patient education and behavior change [90]. Mao et al. evaluated a mobile phone-based health coaching service via app combined with wireless scale, pedometer, and blood pressure cuff on weight loss and blood pressure management among a population of overweight patients. Participants received 4 months of intensive health coaching via live video, phone, and text messages and were also provided with a wireless scale, pedometer, and blood pressure cuff. Among 151 intervention participants with blood pressure data, 112 (74.2%) had a baseline blood pressure that was above the goal (systolic blood pressure > 120 mmHg); 55 out of 112 (49.1%) participants improved their blood pressure at 4 months by an entire hypertensive stage-as defined by the Seventh Report of the Joint National Committee on Prevention, Detection, Evaluation, and Treatment of High Blood Pressure. Participants in the intervention group lost an average of 3.23% total body weight (TBW) at 4 months of coaching and 28.6% (218/763) intervention participants achieved a clinically significant weight loss of 5% or more of TBW, with an average of 9.46% weight loss in this cohort. This suggests that mobile phone app-based health coaching interventions can be an acceptable and effective means to promote blood pressure and weight management in overweight or obese individuals.

Blood Glucose Control Coaching

Earlier, we described various consumer-based tracking systems for blood glucose monitoring. Based on patient self-reports, there is a clear signal of patient interest to streamline glucose monitoring and logging, suggesting that the ability to receive one's own glucose data in a structured manner may improve tracking adherence [91, 92]. A retrospective study by Offringa et al. [93] found that participants who used a mobile platform displaying personalized glucose data in a digital log performed self-monitored glucose checks more frequently and had lower mean glucose levels than controls. Moreover, a systematic review of over 14 trials suggests that mobile applications may provide benefit as an adjuvant to guideline-directed management in patients with type 2 diabetes, with a mean hemoglobin A1c reduction of 0.5% compared to non-users [91]. In a separate systematic review of 12 trials, Wu et al. [92] found that A1c reductions are greater if mobile applications included education on complication prevention, but identified a concern regarding the "decision-making function" featured in 3 mobile applications that provided treatment recommendations derived from an algorithm without clinician oversight. As more patient-facing applications and digital tools enter the market, it is critical that clinicians are involved to oversee algorithm development of any "decision-making" features to prevent adverse health events such as hypoglycemic episodes.

Transformation of Healthcare Delivery

Digital health is positioned to transform health delivery and shape precision medicine practices. Previously in this chapter, we described the role of patient-facing biosensors and software is to generate and collect cardiovascular clinically-relevant data (e.g. heart rate, blood pressure, and biomarkers), detect risk signals, and inform clinicians for health coaching and management. By connecting the streams of health data from the technology-enabled tools with other relevant clinical data the aim is create a multifaceted and highly personalized profile of each patient. Furthermore, the actionable health insights generated from technology-enabled tools will allow for proactive intervention tailored to each individual patient. From a healthcare system architecture standpoint this requires leveraging (1) mobile data capture from patient, (2) secure data platforms, (3) portal for patients to access data and engage with clinicians, and (4) a cloud-connected electronic medical record and/or clinician portal with artificial intelligence capability. In the following schematic overview of telehealth and precision medicine, we illustrate the potential integration among consumer connected health technologies, predictive analytics, and electronic health systems to facilitate clinician decision-making (Fig. 3).

Cardiovascular disease prevention, detection, and management may be more precise, less invasive, and cost-effective as technology adoption increases in the future. In order to do so it will require collaboration between key stakeholders in developing, testing, and implementing the most promising DHIs. Additionally, payers including the US Centers for Medicare & Medicaid Services will play a major role in sustaining technological advancement by adapting regulation and reimbursement policies to support digital services. Ultimately, healthcare organizations and systems will need to systematically identify health technology that

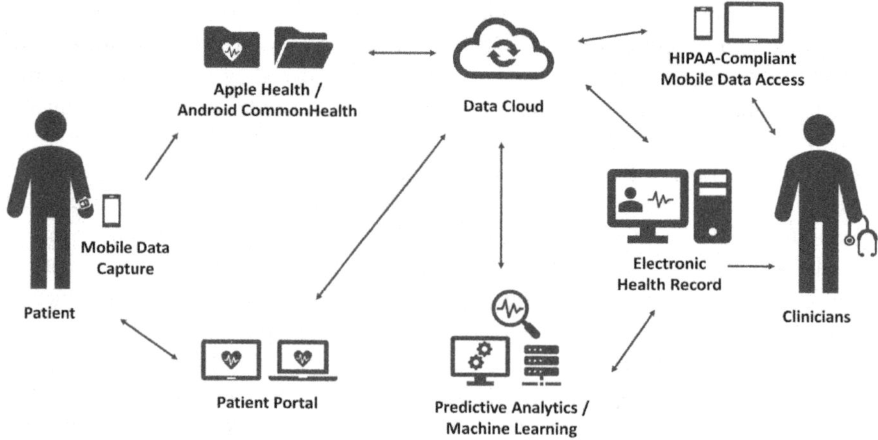

Fig. 3 Digital health data flow and cooperability to enhance precision medicine

offers improvement in clinical care delivery and outcomes in a cost-effective manner. We will provide three examples of how digital health could potentially transform and personalize healthcare delivery in the outpatient clinic, hospital, and post-acute care.

Outpatient Clinic (Chronic Condition Management and Prevention)

The traditional clinic-based office visit is based on a care model which proposes to manage patients with periodic visits and one set of vitals every 3-month, 6-month, 12 month or annual follow-up appointments. A conventional approach such as this is limited by snapshots of the patient's health instead of a holistic and continuous picture. It also creates barriers for access to care including time, costs of travel and parking, absence from work, and is a major barrier to relatively immobile patients. Patients and clinicians are increasingly communicating via HIPAA-compliant electronic patient portals and video-based visits. While these tele-visits are limited by a lack of the physical exam, the benefits of seeing the patient, discussing concerns, and actively tailoring therapy according to transmitted biometric data (e.g. vital signs, step count, weight, biomarkers) have the ability to deepen the patient-clinician relationship. Telemedicine, in addition to promoting health equity by addressing geographic, logistic, and financial barriers to care, is able to leverage technology to individualize care through longitudinal care in the home and community environment. In a highly efficient and modern manner, it can bring medicine back to the days of home visits. This is inherently more personal and patient-centric than hospital based care. Notably, the American Heart Association emphasized a call-to-action for system level changes to improve access to care, citing disparities in rural communities such as a 20% higher mortality rate and 40% higher prevalence rate for CVD compared to urban populations [94] mHealth and telemedicine may be aptly suited to mitigate these disparities by expanding access to care in a cost-efficient manner; further research is necessary to assess the cost-effectiveness and patient outcomes of these interventions.

Inpatient (Acute Care)

The standard hospital discharge process remains problematic for healthcare systems due to multiple handoffs, lack of understanding among patients of care plans, and unacceptable rates of hospital readmission. Individualizing the cardiovascular recovery experience after an acute cardiac event remains a priority for health systems and involves improving the hospital discharge process, transitioning to outpatient management, and promoting long-term adherence to guideline-directed medical therapy. For example, 30-day readmissions for acute myocardial infarction are among the leading causes of preventable morbidity, mortality, and healthcare costs [95]. Digital health interventions may be an effective tool in promoting self-management, adherence to guideline-directed therapy, and cardiovascular risk reduction. One example of how clinicians can leverage mHealth interventions to facilitate the transition from acute inpatient care to long-term outpatient management is the Corrie Health Digital Platform (Corrie) [44]. Corrie is the first cardiology Apple CareKit smartphone application, which is paired with an Apple Watch and iHealth Bluetooth-enabled blood pressure cuff, and was developed to be delivered early in hospitalization for acute myocardial infarction to support guideline-directed medical therapy and prepare patients for post-acute care cardiovascular recovery. The system allows the care team to help set individualized medication logs and patient health information, including care coordination contacts. The Corrie Myocardial infarction, COmbined-device, Recovery Enhancement (MiCORE) study results show reduce all-cause, unplanned 30-day hospital readmissions and related healthcare costs for acute myocardial infarction (AMI) patients.

Case Example of Application of Digital Health Coaching for a Cardiovascular Patient [96]
A 55-year-old woman with undiagnosed familial hypercholesterolemia, pre-diabetes, tobacco use, physical inactivity, diet consisting of fried and processed foods, and morbid obesity was admitted with chest pain. She was diagnosed with an inferior ST-elevation MI and two drug-eluting stents were placed in her right coronary artery. She had previously been incarcerated, earned US$31 000 annually working at a retail store, and had been uninsured

for several years. She had never received preventive care to reduce her cardiac risk factors

While hospitalized, she was enrolled in Corrie Myocardial infarction, Combined-device, Recovery Enhancement (MiCORE) study, which was a trial primarily aimed to determine if type I MI patients using Corrie have lower all-cause unplanned 30-day hospital readmissions and related healthcare costs compared with a historical comparison group. Corrie consists of (1) a smartphone application for medication management, education, vitals and care coordination, (2) cooperative sensors including an Apple Watch and an iHealth wireless blood pressure cuff and (3) a data backend platform. This intervention engages patients early during the hospitalization and facilitates adoption of guideline-directed medical treatment and lifestyle modifications known to improve health outcomes. At the time of enrolment, the patient owned a flip phone and had never used a smartphone. She was provided with an iPhone preloaded with the Corrie app and Apple Watch and wireless blood pressure monitor to participate in the study. She was briefly trained for 30 min on how to use the app, and was provided with an orientation packet highlighting key features of the app

With the help of reminders from the Corrie app on both her phone and watch, she tracked adherence to her cardiac medications and follow-up appointments with her primary care doctor and cardiologist. She monitored her step count and increased her exercise to climbing stairs and/or walking 3–5 miles daily. She learnt more about cardiovascular health and her recent diagnosis through a curriculum consisting of brief, easy to understand and visually engaging educational videos. She also changed her lifestyle, as recommended in the videos, by quitting smoking, avoiding fast and fried foods, eating heart healthy foods and reducing her soda intake by half. At 30 days, and at an interview conducted 2.4 years after initial enrolment, she was continuing healthy daily habits, avoiding both post-MI complications and hospital readmission

Center-Based Services (Post Acute Care)

Cardiac rehabilitation (CR) is an effective modality to reduce cardiovascular mortality and improve health-related quality of life across a broad range of cardiovascular disease (e.g. myocardial Infarction, heart failure, peripheral arterial disease) [97]. CR is a medically supervised program to reinforce guideline-directed medical therapy, risk factor modification, psychosocial support, and exercise training [98]. Despite the strong evidence in support of the benefits of CR, less than 20% of patients who are eligible for CR participate [99]. Low utilization of CR due to lack of time and costs associated with participation and travel, lack of access to a CR facility due to scheduling, transportation, or distance have created an opportunity for a virtual CR model [100].

Digital health technologies have the potential to address the challenges associated with traditional facility-based CR programs with a precision medicine approach by delivering care to patients in the convenience of their own homes and providing real-time, personalized support and individualized activity thresholds. Digital CR is attractive as an adjunct or as an alternative to traditional CR [101–107]. Home- and center-based CR appear similarly effective in improving clinical- and health-related QoL outcomes in myocardial infarction, myocardial revascularization, and heart failure patients [108]. Furthermore, the American Heart Association/American College of Cardiology/American Association of Cardiovascular and Pulmonary Rehabilitation provided a consensus statement highlighting evidence that home- and facility-based CR can achieve similar improvements in 3- to 12-month clinical outcomes [109]. Overall a Virtual Cardiac Rehab transition from traditional facility-based care highlights the potential of telehealth and digital technology to enhance cardiovascular care by broadening access to the evidence-based benefit of CR.

Conclusions

Healthcare is on the verge of a digital health transformation that will deliver the promise of personalized medicine. Health technology can extend cardiovascular expertise to connect cardiologists with patients in resource-limited settings. Stakeholders particularly health consumers, clinicians, innovators, technology industry, payers, and healthcare leadership must forge this pathway together. We share a common purpose to achieve the adoption of digital health and personalized medicine to promote healthier populations, decreased healthcare spending, and improvement in health equity.

The key takeaways from this chapter include understanding:

The role of biosensors, biomarkers, and software that can generate, gather, and share data with clinicians to inform personalized health coaching

How disease could be identified earlier, intervened on proactively, and personalized to the patient to drive their empowerment to execute self-management actions

How healthcare transformation with technology-enabled tools can improve precision medicine across care settings

The importance of advocating to policymakers, payers, insurers, and healthcare administrators for supporting the adoption of health technology.

References

1. Global System for Mobile Communications Association. 'The Mobile Economy 2020. Global System for Mobile Communications Association, London, UK. 2020. https://wwwgsmacom/r/mobileeconomy. Accessed 8 Jan 2020.
2. US Food & Drug Administration. Digital Health. 2020. https://www.fda.gov/medical-devices/digital-health. Accessed 9 Jan 2020.
3. Ryu S. Book review: mHealth: new horizons for health through mobile technologies: based on the findings of the second global survey on eHealth (global observatory for eHealth series, volume 3). Healthcare Inf Res. 2012;18(3):231–3.
4. Steinhubl SR, Muse ED, Topol EJ. The emerging field of mobile health. Sci Transl Med. 2015;7(283):283rv283–283rv283.
5. Smith A, Page D. US smartphone use in 2015. Pew Research Center. 2015;1. https://wwwpewinternetorg/2015/04/01/us-smartphone-use-in-2015/. Accessed 9 January 2020.
6. Khan N, Marvel FA, Wang J, Martin SS. Digital health technologies to promote lifestyle change and adherence. Curr Treatm Opt Cardiovascul Med. 2017;19(8):60.
7. Wongvibulsin S, Martin SS, Steinhubl SR, Muse ED. Connected health technology for cardiovascular disease prevention and management. Curr Treatm Options Cardiovascul Med. 2019;21(6):29.
8. Research2Guidance. Mhealth App Economics 2017: Current Status and Future Trends in Mobile Health. Research 2 Guidance Berlin. 2017. https://research2guidance.com/product/mhealth-economics-2017-current-status-and-future-trends-in-mobile-health/. Accessed 24 Mar 2020.
9. Nicholas J, Shilton K, Schueller SM, Gray EL, Kwasny MJ, Mohr DC. The role of data type and recipient in individuals' perspectives on sharing passively collected smartphone data for mental health: cross-sectional questionnaire study. JMIR mHealth and uHealth. 2019;7(4):e12578.
10. US Food & Drug Administration. Statement from FDA Commissioner Scott Gottlieb, M.D., and Center for Devices and Radiological Health Director Jeff Shuren, M.D., J.D., on agency efforts to work with tech industry to spur innovation in digital health. 2020. https://wwwfdagov/news-events/press-announcements/statement-fda-commissioner-scott-gottlieb-md-and-center-devices-and-radiological-health-director. Accessed 26 Mar 2020.
11. US Food & Drug Administration. Fibricheck Section 510(k) premarket notification. 2018. https://wwwaccessdatafdagov/cdrh_docs/pdf17/K173872pdf. Accessed 25 Mar 2020.
12. US Food & Drug Administration. HeartCheck Cardi Beat ECG Monitor with GEMS Mobile Section 510(k) Premarket Notification. 2019. https://wwwaccessdatafdagov/cdrh_docs/pdf18/K181310pdf. Accessed 25 Mar 2020.
13. US Food & Drug Administration. De Novo Classification Request for Irregular Rhythm Notification Feature. 2018. https://wwwaccessdatafdagov/cdrh_docs/reviews/DEN180042pdf. Accessed 25 Mar 2020.

14. US Food & Drug Administration. De Novo Classification Request For ECG App. 2018. https://wwwaccessdatafdagov/cdrh_docs/reviews/DEN180044pdf. Accessed 25 March 2020.
15. Peerbridge Health Inc. FDA Grants Marketing Clearance For The Peerbridge CorTM Multi-Channel Remote ECG Monitor. 2017. https://wwwpeerbridgehealthcom/fda-grants-marketing-clearance-for-the-peerbridge-cortm-multi-channel-remote-ecg-monitor/. Accessed 25 March 2020.
16. NimbleHeart Inc. FDA clears Physiotrace Smart wearable and reusable device for exercise ECG monitoring. 2017. https://wwwnimbleheartcom/news-page/. Accessed 25 March 2020.
17. AliveCor. FDA grants first ever clearance for six-lead personal ECG device. 2019. https://wwwalivecorcom/press/press_release/fda-grants-first-ever-clearance-for-six-lead-personal-ecg-device/. Accessed 26 March 2020.
18. Al-Alusi MA, Ding E, McManus DD, Lubitz SA. Wearing Your heart on your sleeve: the future of cardiac rhythm monitoring. Curr Cardiol Rep. 2019;21(12):158.
19. Yang WE, Spaulding EM, Lumelsky D, et al. Strategies for the successful implementation of a novel iPhone loaner system (iShare) in mHealth interventions: prospective study. JMIR mHealth and uHealth. 2019;7(12):e16391.
20. Sankari Z, Adeli H. HeartSaver: A mobile cardiac monitoring system for auto-detection of atrial fibrillation, myocardial infarction, and atrio-ventricular block. Comput Biol Med. 2011;41(4):211–20.
21. Turakhia MP. Moving from big data to deep learning—the case of atrial fibrillation. JAMA Cardiol. 2018;3(5):371–2.
22. Koehler F, Koehler K, Deckwart O, et al. Efficacy of telemedical interventional management in patients with heart failure (TIM-HF2): a randomised, controlled, parallel-group, unmasked trial. The Lancet. 2018;392(10152):1047–57.
23. American Heart Association. More than 100 million Americans have high blood pressure, AHA says. 2018. https://wwwheartorg/en/news/2018/05/01/more-than-100-million-americans-have-high-blood-pressure-aha-says. Accessed 26 March 2020.
24. McLean G, Band R, Saunderson K, et al. Digital interventions to promote self-management in adults with hypertension systematic review and meta-analysis. J Hypertens. 2016;34(4):600.
25. Mengden T, Medina RMH, Beltran B, Alvarez E, Kraft K, Vetter H. Reliability of reporting self-measured blood pressure values by hypertensive patients. Am J Hypertens. 1998;11(12):1413–7.
26. McManus RJ, Mant J, Franssen M, et al. Efficacy of self-monitored blood pressure, with or without telemonitoring, for titration of antihypertensive medication (TASMINH4): an unmasked randomised controlled trial. The Lancet. 2018;391(10124):949–59.
27. Tucker KL, Sheppard JP, Stevens R, et al. Self-monitoring of blood pressure in hypertension: a systematic review and individual patient data meta-analysis. PLoS Med. 2017;14(9).
28. Green BB, Cook AJ, Ralston JD, et al. Effectiveness of home blood pressure monitoring, Web communication, and pharmacist care on hypertension control: a randomized controlled trial. JAMA. 2008;299(24):2857–67.
29. Magid DJ, Ho PM, Olson KL, et al. A multimodal blood pressure control intervention in 3 healthcare systems. Am J Manag Care. 2011;17(4):e96-103.
30. Rifkin DE, Abdelmalek JA, Miracle CM, et al. Linking clinic and home: a randomized, controlled clinical effectiveness trial of real-time, wireless blood pressure monitoring for older patients with kidney disease and hypertension. Blood Pres Monit. 2013;18(1):8.
31. Marvel FA, Wang J, Martin SS. Digital health innovation: a toolkit to navigate from concept to clinical testing. JMIR Cardio. 2018;2(1):e2.
32. Hales CM, Carroll MD, Fryar CD, Ogden CL. Prevalence of obesity among adults and youth: United States, 2015–2016. 2017.
33. Cercato C, Fonseca F. Cardiovascular risk and obesity. Diabetol Metab Synd. 2019;11(1):74.

34. National Institute of Health. Executive summary of the clinical guidelines on the identification, evaluation, and treatment of overweight and obesity in adults. Arch Intern Med. 1998;158:1855–67.

35. Blackburn G. Effect of degree of weight loss on health benefits. Obes Res. 1995;3(S2):211s–6s.

36. Nicklas JM, Huskey KW, Davis RB, Wee CC. Successful weight loss among obese US adults. Am J Prev Med. 2012;42(5):481–5.

37. Kraschnewski J, Boan J, Esposito J, et al. Long-term weight loss maintenance in the United States. International J Obes. 2010;34(11):1644–54.

38. Severin R, Sabbahi A, Mahmoud AM, Arena R, Phillips SA. Precision medicine in weight loss and healthy living. Prog Cardiovasc Dis. 2019;62(1):15–20.

39. Yanovski SZ, Yanovski JA. Long-term drug treatment for obesity: a systematic and clinical review. JAMA. 2014;311(1):74–86.

40. Bhagat YA, Kim I, Choi A, Kim JY, Jo S, Cho J. Mind your composition: clinical validation of Samsung's pocket-based bioelectrical impedance analyzers may increase consumer interest in personal health management. IEEE Pulse. 2015;6(5):20–5.

41. Cohen MJ, Shaykevich S, Cawthon C, Kripalani S, Paasche-Orlow MK, Schnipper JL. Predictors of medication adherence postdischarge: the impact of patient age, insurance status, and prior adherence. J Hosp Med. 2012;7(6):470–5.

42. Jha AK, Aubert RE, Yao J, Teagarden JR, Epstein RS. Greater adherence to diabetes drugs is linked to less hospital use and could save nearly $5 billion annually. Health Aff. 2012;31(8):1836–46.

43. Conway CM, Kelechi TJ. Digital health for medication adherence in adult diabetes or hypertension: an integrative review. JMIR Diab. 2017;2(2):e20.

44. Spaulding EM, Marvel FA, Lee MA, et al. Corrie health digital platform for self-management in secondary prevention after acute myocardial infarction. Circul Cardiovascul Quality Outcomes. 2019;12(5):e005509.

45. Granger BB, Locke SC, Bowers M, et al. The digital drag and drop pillbox: design and feasibility of a skill-based education model to improve medication management. J Cardiovascul Nurs. 2017;32(5):E14.

46. Browne SH, Peloquin C, Santillo F, et al. Digitizing medicines for remote capture of oral medication adherence using co-encapsulation. Clin Pharmacol Ther. 2018;103(3):502–10.

47. Van Biesen W, Decruyenaere J, Sideri K, Cockbain J, Sterckx S. Remote digital monitoring of medication intake: methodological, medical, ethical and legal reflections. Acta Clinica Belgica. 2019:1–8.

48. Martin SS, Feldman DI, Blumenthal RS, et al. mActive: a randomized clinical trial of an automated mHealth intervention for physical activity promotion. J Am Heart Assoc. 2015;4(11):e002239.

49. Compernolle S, Vandelanotte C, Cardon G, De Bourdeaudhuij I, De Cocker K. Effectiveness of a web-based, computer-tailored, pedometer-based physical activity intervention for adults: a cluster randomized controlled trial. J Med Internet Res. 2015;17(2):e38.

50. Cheatham SW, Stull KR, Fantigrassi M, Motel I. The efficacy of wearable activity tracking technology as part of a weight loss program: a systematic review. J Sports Med Phys Fit. 2018;58(4):534–48.

51. Finkelstein EA, Haaland BA, Bilger M, et al. Effectiveness of activity trackers with and without incentives to increase physical activity (TRIPPA): a randomised controlled trial. Lancet Diab Endocrinol. 2016;4(12):983–95.

52. Zaidan S, Roehrer E. Popular mobile phone apps for diet and weight loss: a content analysis. JMIR mHealth and uHealth. 2016;4(3):e80.

53. Dunn CG, Turner-McGrievy GM, Wilcox S, Hutto B. Dietary self-monitoring through calorie tracking but not through a digital photography app is associated with significant weight loss: The 2SMART pilot study—A 6-month randomized trial. J Acad Nutr Diet. 2019;119(9):1525–32.

54. Ferrara G, Kim J, Lin S, Hua J, Seto E. A focused review of smartphone diet-tracking apps: usability, functionality, coherence with behavior change theory, and comparative validity of nutrient intake and energy estimates. JMIR mHealth and uHealth. 2019;7(5):e9232.

55. Oktay AA, Akturk HK, Esenboğa K, Javed F, Polin NM, Jahangir E. Pathophysiology and prevention of heart disease in diabetes mellitus. Curr Probl Cardiol. 2018;43(3):68–110.

56. Preis SR, Hwang S-J, Coady S, et al. Trends in all-cause and cardiovascular disease mortality among women and men with and without diabetes in the Framingham Heart Study, 1950–2005. Circulation. 2009;119(13):1728.

57. Schramm T, Gislasson G, Kober L, Rasmussen S, Rasmussen J, Abildstrom S. Diabetes patients requiring glucosa-lowerin therapy and nondiabetics with a prior myocardial infarction carry the same cardiovascular risk. A Population Study of 3.3 million people. Circulation. 2008;117:1945–1954.

58. Selvin E, Marinopoulos S, Berkenblit G, et al. Meta-analysis: glycosylated hemoglobin and cardiovascular disease in diabetes mellitus. Ann Intern Med. 2004;141(6):421–31.

59. Gerstein H, Islam S, Anand S, et al. Dysglycaemia and the risk of acute myocardial infarction in multiple ethnic groups: an analysis of 15,780 patients from the INTERHEART study. Diabetologia. 2010;53(12):2509–17.

60. Association AD. 6. Glycemic targets: standards of medical care in diabetes—2018. *Diabetes Care.* 2018;41(Supplement 1):S55–S64.

61. Segman Y. Device and method for noninvasive glucose assessment. J Diabetes Sci Technol. 2018;12(6):1159–68.

62. Lee H, Song C, Hong YS, et al. Wearable/disposable sweat-based glucose monitoring device with multistage transdermal drug delivery module. Sci Advan. 2017;3(3):e1601314.

63. Woldaregay AZ, Årsand E, Walderhaug S, et al. Data-driven modeling and prediction of blood glucose dynamics: machine learning applications in type 1 diabetes. Artificial intelligence in medicine. 2019.

64. Olafsdottir AF, Attvall S, Sandgren U, et al. A clinical trial of the accuracy and treatment experience of the flash glucose monitor FreeStyle Libre in adults with type 1 diabetes. Diabetes Technology & Therapeutics. 2017;19(3):164–72.

65. Bidonde J, Fagerlund BC, Frønsdal KB, Lund UH, Robberstad B. FreeStyle libre flash glucose self-monitoring system: a single-technology assessment. 2017.

66. Abraham WT, Stevenson LW, Bourge RC, Lindenfeld JA, Bauman JG, Adamson PB, CHAMPION Trial Study Group. Sustained efficacy of pulmonary artery pressure to guide adjustment of chronic heart failure therapy: complete follow-up results from the CHAMPION randomised trial. The Lancet. 2016 Jan 30;387(10017):453–61.

67. US Food & Drug Administration. CardioMEMS™ HF System. Summary of Safety and Effectiveness Data. Available at: https://www.accessdata.fda.gov/cdrh_docs/pdf10/P100045b.pdf. Accessed 17 Jun 2020.

68. Painter JE, Borba CP, Hynes M, Mays D, Glanz K. The use of theory in health behavior research from 2000 to 2005: a systematic review. Ann Behav Med. 2008;35(3):358–62.

69. Rosenstock IM. Historical origins of the health belief model. Health Edu Monog. 1974;2(4):328–35.

70. Glanz K, Bishop DB. The role of behavioral science theory in development and implementation of public health interventions. Annu Rev Public Health. 2010;31:399–418.

71. Will JC, Farris RP, Sanders CG, Stockmyer CK, Finkelstein EA. Health promotion interventions for disadvantaged women: overview of the WISEWOMAN projects. J Women's Health. 2004;13(5):484–502.

72. Query ID="Q1' Text="Unable to parse this reference. Kindly do manual structure' Bandura A. Social foundations of thought and action. Englewood Cliffs, NJ. 1986;1986.

73. Ammerman AS, Lindquist CH, Lohr KN, Hersey J. The efficacy of behavioral interventions to modify dietary fat and fruit and vegetable intake: a review of the evidence. Prev Med. 2002;35(1):25–41.

74. Legler J, Meissner HI, Coyne C, Breen N, Chollette V, Rimer BK. The effectiveness of interventions to promote mammography among women with historically lower rates of screening. Cancer Epidemiol Prevent Biomark. 2002;11(1):59–71.
75. Noar SM, Benac CN, Harris MS. Does tailoring matter? Meta-analytic review of tailored print health behavior change interventions. Psychol Bull. 2007;133(4):673.
76. Taylor N, Conner M, Lawton R. The impact of theory on the effectiveness of worksite physical activity interventions: a meta-analysis and meta-regression. Health Psychol Rev. 2012;6(1):33–73.
77. Webb T, Joseph J, Yardley L, Michie S. Using the internet to promote health behavior change: a systematic review and meta-analysis of the impact of theoretical basis, use of behavior change techniques, and mode of delivery on efficacy. J Med Internet Res. 2010;12(1):e4.
78. Lyons EJ, Lewis ZH, Mayrsohn BG, Rowland JL. Behavior change techniques implemented in electronic lifestyle activity monitors: a systematic content analysis. J Med Internet Res. 2014;16(8):e192.
79. Lewis ZH, Lyons EJ, Jarvis JM, Baillargeon J. Using an electronic activity monitor system as an intervention modality: a systematic review. BMC Public Health. 2015;15(1):585.
80. Black N, Johnston M, Michie S, et al. Behaviour Change techniques associated with smoking cessation in intervention and comparator groups of randomised controlled trials: a systematic review and meta-regression. *Addiction*.n/a(n/a).
81. Abroms LC, Boal AL, Simmens SJ, Mendel JA, Windsor RA. A randomized trial of Text2Quit: a text messaging program for smoking cessation. Am J Prev Med. 2014;47 (3):242–50.
82. Robinson CD, Wiseman KP, Webb Hooper M, et al. Engagement and short-term abstinence outcomes among blacks and whites in the national cancer institute's smokefreeTXT program. Nicotine & Tobacco Research. 2019.
83. Müssener U, Bendtsen M, Karlsson N, White IR, McCambridge J, Bendtsen P. Effectiveness of short message service text-based smoking cessation intervention among university students: a randomized clinical trial. JAMA Inter Med. 2016;176(3):321–8.
84. Liao Y, Wu Q, Kelly BC, et al. Effectiveness of a text-messaging-based smoking cessation intervention ("Happy Quit") for smoking cessation in China: a randomized controlled trial. PLoS Med. 2018;15(12).
85. Spohr SA, Nandy R, Gandhiraj D, Vemulapalli A, Anne S, Walters ST. Efficacy of SMS text message interventions for smoking cessation: a meta-analysis. J Subst Abuse Treat. 2015;56:1–10.
86. Naughton F. Delivering, "Just-In-Time" smoking cessation support via mobile phones: current knowledge and future directions. Nicotine Tob Res. 2017;19(3):379–83.
87. Struik LL, Baskerville NB. The role of facebook in crush the crave, a mobile-and social media-based smoking cessation intervention: qualitative framework analysis of posts. J Med Internet Res. 2014;16(7):e170.
88. Benjamin EJ, Virani SS, Callaway CW, et al. Forecasting the future of cardiovascular disease in the United States: a policy statement from the American Heart Association. Circulation. 2018;137(12):e67–492.
89. Uhlig K, Patel K, Ip S, Kitsios GD, Balk EM. Self-measured blood pressure monitoring in the management of hypertension: a systematic review and meta-analysis. Ann Intern Med. 2013;159(3):185–94.
90. Mao AY, Chen C, Magana C, Caballero Barajas K, Olayiwola JN. A mobile phone-based health coaching intervention for weight loss and blood pressure reduction in a national payer population: a retrospective study. JMIR mHealth and uHealth. 2017;5(6):e80.
91. Hou C, Carter B, Hewitt J, Francisa T, Mayor S. Do mobile phone applications improve glycemic control (HbA1c) in the self-management of diabetes? A systematic review, meta-analysis, and GRADE of 14 randomized trials. Diabetes Care. 2016;39(11):2089–95.
92. Wu Y, Yao X, Vespasiani G, et al. Mobile app-based interventions to support diabetes self-management: a systematic review of randomized controlled trials to identify functions associated with glycemic efficacy. JMIR mHealth and uHealth. 2017;5(3):e35.

93. Offringa R, Sheng T, Parks L, Clements M, Kerr D, Greenfield MS. Digital diabetes management application improves glycemic outcomes in people with type 1 and type 2 diabetes. J Diabetes Sci Technol. 2018;12(3):701–8.

94. Harrington RA, Califf RM, Balamurugan A, et al. Call to action: rural health: a presidential advisory from the American heart association and American stroke association. Circulation. 2020;141(10):e615–44.

95. Hines A, Barrett M, Jiang HJ, Steiner C. Conditions with the largest number of adult hospital readmissions by payer, 2011: statistical brief# 172. 2006.

96. Hung G, Yang WE, Marvel FA, Martin SS. Mobile health application platform 'Corrie'personalises and empowers the heart attack recovery patient experience in the hospital and at home for an underserved heart attack survivor. BMJ Case Reports CP. 2020;13(2).

97. Anderson L, Oldridge N, Thompson DR, et al. Exercise-based cardiac rehabilitation for coronary heart disease: cochrane systematic review and meta-analysis. J Am Coll Cardiol. 2016;67(1):1–12.

98. Balady GJ, Williams MA, Ades PA, et al. Core components of cardiac rehabilitation/ secondary prevention programs: 2007 update: a scientific statement from the American heart association exercise, cardiac rehabilitation, and prevention committee, the council on clinical cardiology; the councils on cardiovascular nursing, epidemiology and prevention, and nutrition, physical activity, and metabolism; and the American association of cardiovascular and pulmonary rehabilitation. Circulation. 2007;115(20):2675–82.

99. Boyden T, Rubenfire M, Franklin B. Will increasing referral to cardiac rehabilitation improve participation? Prevent Cardiol. 2010;13(4):192–201.

100. Balady GJ, Ades PA, Bittner VA, et al. Referral, enrollment, and delivery of cardiac rehabilitation/secondary prevention programs at clinical centers and beyond: a presidential advisory from the American heart association. Circulation. 2011;124(25):2951–60.

101. Pfaeffli Dale L, Whittaker R, Jiang Y, Stewart R, Rolleston A, Maddison R. Text message and internet support for coronary heart disease self-management: results from the text4heart randomized controlled trial. J Med Internet Res. 2015;17(10):e237.

102. Varnfield M, Karunanithi M, Lee CK, et al. Smartphone-based home care model improved use of cardiac rehabilitation in postmyocardial infarction patients: results from a randomised controlled trial. Heart (British Cardiac Society). 2014;100(22):1770–9.

103. Maddison R, Rawstorn JC, Stewart RAH, et al. Effects and costs of real-time cardiac telerehabilitation: randomised controlled non-inferiority trial. Heart (British Cardiac Society). 2019;105(2):122–9.

104. Fang J, Huang B, Xu D, Li J, Au WW. Innovative application of a home-based and remote sensing cardiac rehabilitation protocol in Chinese patients after percutaneous coronary intervention. Telemed J E-Health Off J Am Telemed Assoc. 2019;25(4):288–93.

105. Peng X, Su Y, Hu Z, et al. Home-based telehealth exercise training program in Chinese patients with heart failure: a randomized controlled trial. Medicine. 2018;97(35):e12069.

106. Forman DE, LaFond K, Panch T, Allsup K, Manning K, Sattelmair J. Utility and efficacy of a smartphone application to enhance the learning and behavior goals of traditional cardiac rehabilitation: a feasibility study. J Cardiopul Rehabil Preven. 2014;34(5):327–34.

107. Piotrowicz E, Baranowski R, Bilinska M, et al. A new model of home-based telemonitored cardiac rehabilitation in patients with heart failure: effectiveness, quality of life, and adherence. Eur J Heart Fail. 2010;12(2):164–71.

108. Anderson L, Sharp GA, Norton RJ, et al. Home-based versus centre-based cardiac rehabilitation. Cochrane Database Syst Rev. 2017;6:Cd007130.

109. Thomas RJ, Beatty AL, Beckie TM, et al. Home-based cardiac rehabilitation: a scientific statement from the american association of cardiovascular and pulmonary rehabilitation, the American heart association, and the American college of cardiology. J Am Coll Cardiol. 2019;74(1):133–53.

Artificial Intelligence and Machine Learning

Fawzi Zghyer, Sharan Yadav, and Mohamed B. Elshazly

The greatest opportunity offered by AI is not reducing errors or workloads, or even curing cancer: it is the opportunity to restore the precious and time-honored connection and trust— the human touch—between patients and doctors.

—Eric Topol

Preventive Cardiology, the Past and the Future

Cardiologists, for many years, have been successful in implementing measures and pioneering medical therapies and interventions to treat cardiovascular diseases. These measures have become very advanced and aggressive; however, accurate risk assessment and prevention promise to have the biggest impact on the human health span. Continuous renovation of primary and secondary prevention strategies is needed now more than ever [1, 2] as we shift towards a new era of big data and personalized interventions leading to the democratization of medicine.

Risk prediction is the foundation of prevention, and the Framingham studies set the stage for Atherosclerotic Cardiovascular Disease (ASCVD) risk prediction using clinical scores. Other primary prevention cohorts such as the Atherosclerosis Risk in Communities study (ARIC) and the Multi-Ethnic study of Atherosclerosis (MESA) [3, 4] have helped further refine risk scores over the years and new

F. Zghyer
Department of Medicine, Johns Hopkins Hospital, Baltimore, MD, USA

S. Yadav · M. B. Elshazly (✉)
Department of Medicine, Weill Cornell Medicine, New York, NY, USA
e-mail: mes2015@qatar-med.cornell.edu

M. B. Elshazly
Department of Medical Education, Weill Cornell Medicine, Doha, Qatar

Ciccarone Center for the Prevention of Cardiovascular Disease, Johns Hopkins University School of Medicine, Baltimore, MD, USA

© Springer Nature Switzerland AG 2021
S. S. Martin (ed.), *Precision Medicine in Cardiovascular Disease Prevention,*
https://doi.org/10.1007/978-3-030-75055-8_6

markers such as C-reactive protein and Coronary Artery Calcium (CAC) have been suggested as risk modifiers. However, the core of risk assessment strategies has not significantly changed. Clinical risk scores are not dynamic enough, lack granularity, do not incorporate important information such as lifestyle behaviors and polygenic risk, and are not very accurate at predicting lifelong risk, which is essential for primordial prevention. Moreover, other cardiovascular diseases such as heart failure (HF) or atrial fibrillation do not have well-developed risk assessment scores.

Advancements in technology and big data collection and analysis will undoubtedly allow us to identify more risk factors for cardiovascular diseases. With the increased availability of personalized lifestyle and pharmacotherapeutic interventions, the science and field of prevention are evolving at a great pace. The future of cardiovascular disease prevention will involve the use of dynamic real-world patient data collected from lifestyle surveys or chatbots, smart wearables, or imaging studies coupled with genomics, demographics and clinical risk factors; all trained and continuously fine-tuned by evolving and personalized artificial intelligence (AI) algorithms.

Artificial Intelligence, Machine Learning, and Deep Learning

Widespread digitization and abundance of data has led to machine learning and AI analytical skills becoming some of the most sought-after skills today. AI, which has been around since the 1950s, is the study of intelligent agents that perceive their environment and act accordingly to maximize the chances of successfully achieving their goals [5]. Machine Learning (ML), a form of AI, is a characterized software that can progressively learn from data and make predictions without explicit prior programming [6]. ML can be used to analyze large amounts of data, making it particularly useful for tasks requiring automation.

ML algorithms can be trained via supervised, unsupervised, semi-supervised, reinforcement, and active learning tasks (Fig. 1) [7]. Most of the studies that will be discussed in this chapter utilize supervised learning algorithms. This involves learning a function, through a labeled training dataset where both input and desired output data are provided [8]. After sufficient training, the ML system can then perform the tasks on unlabeled input data. Linear regression, logistic regression, decision tree, random forest, support vector machine, and deep neural networks are some commonly employed supervised learning algorithms [8]. In contrast, in unsupervised learning, algorithms are provided with input data without corresponding output values [8]. The focus is on detecting patterns in a data set, making it popular in applications of clustering, association, or predicting rules that describe a data set [9]. Examples of unsupervised learning algorithms include k-means clustering, hierarchical clustering and principal component analysis [8]. Both semi-supervised learning and active learning involve partially labelled input data [8].

Deep learning (DL), which involves algorithms called artificial neural networks (ANNs) that are inspired by the structure and function of the brain, is a part of the broader family of ML. It involves computational models composed of multiple processing layers, consisting of interconnected "nodes" analogous to neurons in the brain [8]. Some noteworthy classes of DL architecture include deep neural network (DNN), convolutional neural network (CNN), and recurrent neural network (RNN) [10].

There has been growing interest in utilizing AI and ML in healthcare, and it has already been demonstrated to be helpful in a variety of different areas of medicine including cancer diagnosis [11], imaging, and drug development [12], to name a few. Cardiology is one of the fields that can benefit from utilization of this technology. Although AI has mostly been used in imaging thus far, its ability to efficiently analyze large amounts of data make it promising for several aspects of patient care. Research has been done to apply ML in cardiology to imaging, electrocardiography, in-hospital telemonitoring, and mobile and wearable technology [8]. In the era of precision medicine, ML can be applied to the early diagnosis and development of patient tailored therapies, and in the prediction of different cardiovascular diseases [13] (Figs. 1 and 2).

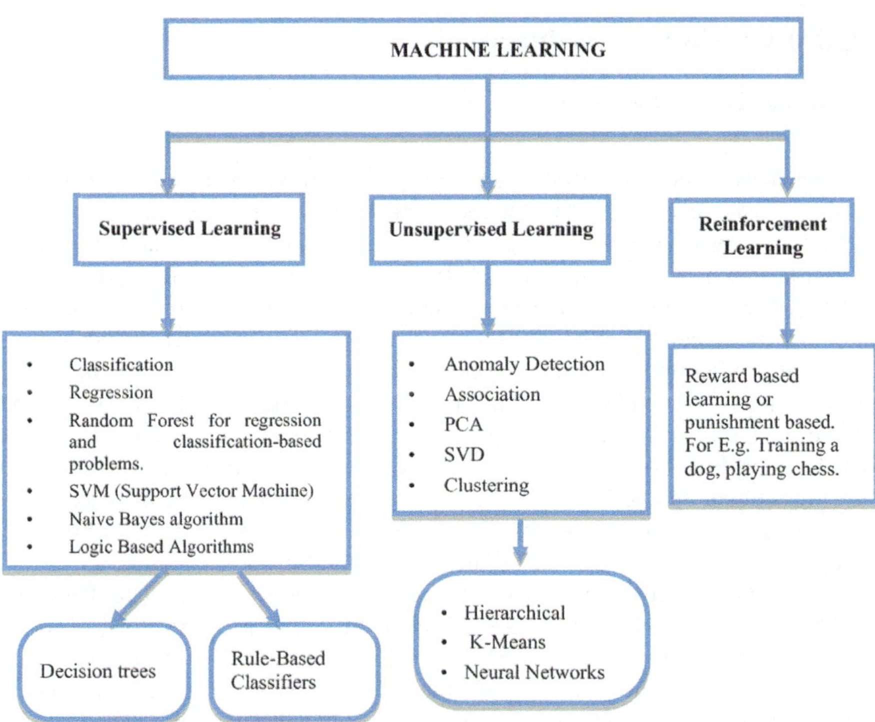

Fig. 1 Machine learning algorithms. Adopted from Springer Nature Media [72]

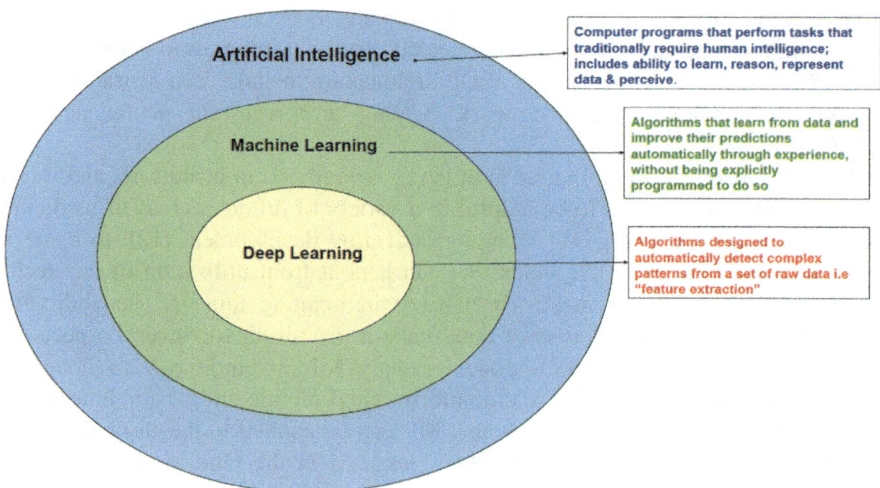

Fig. 2 Artificial intelligence, Machine learning, and Deep learning

Applications in the Cardiovascular Care

Coronary Artery Disease

Approximately every 40 seconds an American will suffer from a myocardial infarction. This year ~720,000 Americans will have a new coronary event [14]. Despite the advancements in diagnostic strategies and primary and secondary prevention, coronary artery disease (CAD) remains a major source of morbidity and mortality. Our current methods of estimating ASCVD risk involve incorporating traditional risk factors to predict the risk of events over a defined period of time [16]. Event prediction is crucial to the current practice of cardiology, as it allows for characterization of sub-clinical disease processes, modification of risk factors and primordial or primary prevention. 10-year risk calculators such as the ACC/AHA Pooled Cohort Equation, though beneficial in practice, tend to underestimate CVD events in women and certain ethnic groups, and overestimate risk in others [17]. There remains a need to develop more accurate tools for early detection of high-risk groups, and this is where ML techniques show promise.

Several studies have developed ML-based techniques using data from the Multi-ethnic study of atherosclerosis (MESA). MESA is a prospective, observational cohort study that included 6814 participants aged 45–84, representing four racial/ethnic groups, who were free of clinical cardiovascular disease at enrollment [18]. Baseline examinations were extensive and included measurement of CAC using computed tomography, cardiac MRI measurement of ventricular mass, ankle and brachial blood pressure, and ECGs among others. Baseline microalbuminuria, standard cardiovascular risk factors, lifestyle habits, and psychosocial factors were also collected. Participants were observed over a median of more than 10 years for identification and characterization of cardiovascular events, including myocardial infarction, stroke, peripheral vascular disease, HF, and mortality, in addition to characterization of therapeutic interventions initiated over the years [18]. For the duration of the study, measurements of selected subclinical disease indicators and risk factors were repeated. Kakadiaris et al. developed an ML based risk calculator utilizing Support Vector Machines (SVMs) on a 13-year follow up data set from MESA, and compared their results to the ACC/AHA Risk Calculator [19]. SVM's are supervised learning algorithms that are fine-tuned by human experts in the field. The FLEMENGHO study served as an external cohort for validation. Their proposed calculator utilized the same 9 traditional risk factors as the ACC/AHA Calculator. Yet, despite having identical inputs, it outperformed the ACC/AHA Calculator by detecting 13% more high-risk individuals and 25% more low-risk individuals who may not need statin therapy [19]. Moreover, the ML Risk Calculator was successful at predicting both "Hard" and "All" cardiovascular events, and performed well in males and females. Ambale-Venkatesh and colleagues also utilized data from MESA, using a random survival forests (RF) technique to identify the top 20 predictors of each endpoint in the study [20]. They found that imaging, ECG, and serum biomarkers featured more heavily than traditional CV risk factors. Age was noted to be the most important predictor for all-cause mortality, while CAC score was the most important predictor of coronary heart disease and all ASCVD combined [20]. The proposed RF technique outperformed established risk scores with increased prediction accuracy.

CAC score from routine cardiac-gated non-contrast CT scans is frequently used in addition to traditional risk factors to enhance cardiovascular risk prediction. Al'Aref et al. developed an ML model incorporating CAC score, in addition to clinical and demographic factors, to predict the presence of obstructive CAD on Cardiac Computed Tomographic Angiography (CCTA). They screened the CONFIRM registry to select 13,054 participants who were evaluated with CCTA for suspected or previously established CAD. They used a boosted ensemble algorithm, a method that combines several decision trees classifiers to produce a more accurate predictive model [21]. They compared the performance of the ML model with and without CAC score, the CAD consortium clinical score alone and with CAC score, and the updated Diamond-Forrester score. ML incorporating the CAC score had the best performance with an AUC of 0.881, and CAC, age, and gender were the highest-ranking features. Such an approach can improve risk stratification and guide management. Han et al. used an ML framework to integrate CCTA derived quantitative and qualitative plaque features to predict those at risk for rapid coronary plaque progression (RPP) [22]. RPP, defined as the annual progression of atheroma percentage volume by $\geq 1.0\%$, is associated with incident cardiovascular events [22]. The study utilized data from 1083 patients in the PARADIGM registry. They designed three different ML models including combinations of clinical features, qualitative, and quantitative plaque characteristics, and compared them to the ACC/AHA pooled cohort equation, Duke coronary artery disease score, and a logistic regression statistical model. The ML model incorporating clinical, qualitative, and quantitative plaque features, had the highest discriminatory performance to identify those at risk for RPP, with quantitative atherosclerosis being the most important feature [22].

CCTA based risk stratification traditionally relies on detecting obstructive lesions or coronary calcification. However, Oikonomou et al. took a different approach to risk prediction by using AI to analyze the radiomic profile of coronary perivascular adipose tissue (PVAT) [23]. Vascular inflammation is now known to cause spatial shifts in PVAT composition, captured by the perivascular Fat Attenuation Index (FAI) [24]. FAI has been shown to have prognostic value for all cause and cardiac cause mortality, however it may lose its prognostic value in patients on appropriate pharmacotherapy [25]. Using ML, they were able to build a new radiomic signature of high-risk PVAT, namely the perivascular Fat Radiomic Profile, that relies on detection of more persistent structural changes associated with PVAT fibrosis and microvascular remodeling induced by chronic coronary inflammation. They verified their method in three different studies, and trained the algorithm to identify those at risk for major adverse cardiac events (MACE). Applying their method to the SCOT-HEART trial significantly improved MACE prediction beyond traditional risk stratification that included risk factors, CAC, coronary stenosis, and high-risk plaque features on CCTA [23]. This study illustrates how ML, when applied to imaging, can help identify new patterns of significant clinical value. The authors of the study propose a 'radio-transcriptomic' approach by linking such imaging patterns to underlying tissue biology and gene expression status. This could lead to more granular and individualized assessment of disease activity and provide novel insights into pathogenesis [23].

The advent of precision medicine relies in part on the availability of accurate and predictive polygenic risk scores. The cost of sequencing the human genome is rapidly decreasing, allowing for development of genomic risk prediction models accessible to the entire population. ML can be utilized to this end due to its capacity to integrate a large number of predictors. Pare et al. developed an ML-based technique to boost the predictive performance of polygenic risk scores using gradient boosted regression trees, leading to significant improvements in the predictive ability (R^2) of risk scores [26]. Okser et al. searched for subsets of genetic variants and their interactions that are most predictive of the various risk classes for atherosclerosis. They developed a predictive model using Single Nucleotide Polymorphisms (SNPs) selected via ML, combined with clinical risk factors, to predict the extreme classes of risk for atherosclerosis and progression over a 6-year period [27]. They achieved AUCs of 0.84 and 0.76 for the risk prediction and disease progressions tasks, respectively, which were both significantly better than those achieved using conventional risk factors alone [27].

Nevertheless, some of the parameters utilized in ML risk scores described above may not be readily available to clinicians, and imaging studies can be time consuming. Poplin et al. were thus interested in extracting signals for cardiovascular risk from retinal images, which can be obtained quickly, cheaply and non-invasively in an outpatient setting. They trained deep learning models to make quantitative predictions of popular cardiovascular risk factors from retinal fundus images from the UK Biobank and EyePACS, and tested their models on images from these databases [28]. The proposed models were found to predict the smoking status with an AUC of 0.71, systolic BP with a mean absolute error within 11.23 mm Hg (95% CI, 11.18–11.51), and MACE with an AUC of 0.70 [28]. The prediction of MACE achieved a comparable accuracy to the SCORE risk calculator [28]. Wang et al. also applied deep learning techniques, using CNNs to discriminate breast arterial calcification (BAC) from non–BAC on mammograms [29]. The free-response ROC analysis of their model showed a level of detection similar to the human experts [29]. Since breast arterial calcification has been proposed as a risk indicator for CAD, stroke, and HF [30], these results are promising for development of an automated system for BAC detection and cardiovascular risk assessment in women undergoing mammograms.

Heart Failure

HF has a high prevalence, affecting around 2% of the adult population in developed countries, including >6.2 million Americans above the age of 20 [31]. Its prevalence is rising, along with the associated morbidity, mortality, and increasing healthcare costs. Thus, early accurate diagnosis and estimation of the severity of HF is crucial. Currently, clinical decision algorithms used to diagnose HF in non-acute settings utilize pertinent clinical history, physical examination, ECG data, along with labs such as Brain Natriuretic Peptide (BNP) to identify patients requiring an echocardiogram. There are several studies that have looked at using ML techniques to detect the presence or absence of HF, making diagnosis more efficient. Most reported studies utilize short or long-term heart rate variability (HRV) incorporated within ML algorithms such as SVMs, decision trees or neural networks, to classify patients as having or not having HF. For example, Melillo et al. studied the discrimination power of long-term HRV measures for diagnosis of chronic HF, using a decision tree method known as CART [32]. Their classification scheme achieved a sensitivity of 89.74%, and a specificity of 100%. Similar results have been obtained in other studies looking at long term [33], as well as short term, HRV [34, 35]. A 2014 study by Liu et al. utilized three nonstandard short-term HRV features in an SVM based HF classification model, and achieved accuracy values of 100% [36]. These results are promising given the rising popularity of smartphones and wearable devices with capabilities for HR monitoring.

Studies have also looked at the risk of developing HF by considering factors other HRV. Aljaaf et al. proposed multi-level risk assessment for developing HF, where patients were classified into 5 categories of increasing risk using a decision tree classifier. The algorithm was trained using the Cleveland Clinic heart disease dataset with three additional risk factors—obesity, physical activity and smoking—achieving an overall precision of 86% [37]. Others, such as Yang et al., suggested a scoring method which allows both the detection of HF as well as assessment of its severity [38]. They also classified the non-HF patients to a Healthy group or to a HF-prone group. The model achieved a total accuracy of 74% [38]. Zheng et al. proposed an innovative Least Squares SVM based model that utilized heart sounds and cardiac reserve features to diagnose HF, achieving diagnostic accuracy, sensitivity and specificity of 95%, 97% and 94% respectively [39]. RNNs, which can take the temporal relationships between different clinical events into consideration, have been successfully employed in some studies. Choi et al. focused on predicting the onset of HF by applying RNNs to longitudinal structured patient data such as diagnosis, medication, and procedure codes in electronic health records [40].

In addition to diagnosis and risk prediction, ML techniques can help in identification of novel risk factors for HF. A recent study applied ML to the UK biobank sample of 500,451 individuals, excluding those with prior HF. Patients were followed up for 9.8 years. Leg bio-impedance was noted to be lower in those who developed HF, and after adjusting for known HF risk factors, was shown to be inversely related to HF [41]. The authors created a model including leg bio-impedance, sex, age, history of myocardial infarction that showed good discrimination for future HF hospitalization (Concordance index = 0.82) [41].

Atrial Fibrillation

Atrial fibrillation (AF) is the most common cardiac arrhythmia globally. Currently, there are 2.2 million cases in the US [42]. AF is an arrhythmia with a propensity towards the ageing population; the prevalence of AF is 0.5% in individuals aged 50–59, but can go up to 10% in individuals aged 80–89 [43]. Interestingly, it is estimated that up to 40% of AF patients will go on undiagnosed [44]. While AF itself is not life threatening, patients are at an increased risk for thromboembolic events, particularly strokes that result in a great deal of morbidity and mortality [45]. Earlier diagnosis of AF and treatment with anticoagulation significantly decreases the risk of strokes [46, 47].

While a 12 lead ECG can be used to check for the presence of AF, it is just analogous to a random blood glucose in the diagnosis of diabetes. A more comprehensive window like glycated hemoglobin is needed for accurate diagnosis especially in patients with paroxysmal AF (PAF). Currently, prolonged ambulatory rhythm monitoring is used to screen for the presence of AF, especially following a stroke [48]. Prolonged monitoring with traditional devices such as Holter monitors is cumbersome, costly, and not of great yield. More advanced automated techniques using traditional ECG or wearable devices combined with ML will become the future of AF prediction and diagnosis.

Attia et al. were among the first to use CNNs to identify the electrocardiographic signature of AF present during normal sinus rhythm. They used an AI model to pinpoint ECG signals, that might be invisible to the human eye but contain important information about the presence of AF. The AI was trained solely using the usual 12 lead 10-s ECG strip and included 180,922 patients and 649,931 normal sinus rhythm ECGs. In their study, they found that the AI model performed well with an area under the curve (AUC) of 0.87 for a single lead ECG and 0.90 for multiple leads in detecting AF [49]. This performs better compared to other medical screening tests such as B-natriuretic peptide for HF with an AUC of 0.6–0.70 [50] as well as CHA_2DS_2-VASc score for stroke risk in AF with an AUC of 0.57–0.72 [51]. Attia and colleagues were successful in showing the power of advanced computer technology, non-linear models, large datasets as well as the use of convolutional neural layers in the diagnosis of a prevalent disease [49].

The Apple Heart Study utilized a commercial smart wearable device, an Apple watch Model 3 or earlier model without ECG, to screen for AF using photoplethysmography tachograms and AF notification algorithms. The group used the irregular pulse notification algorithm, which if activated, would initiate a telemedicine visit and then an ECG patch would be sent to the participant to be worn for 7 days. The possibility of receiving an irregular pulse notification was low at 0.52%. Among the participants who received an irregular pulse notification, 34% had an irregular pulse on subsequent ECG monitoring, and 84% of the irregular pulse notifications were concordant with atrial fibrillation [15].

In another study published by Tiwari and colleagues, the group explored if machine learning can be applied to electronic health record (EHR) data to identify patients at risk of 6-month incident AF. The study used data from 2,252,219 patients, of which 28,037 (1.2%) developed AF at the end of the 6 months interval. In their investigation of the application of an ML model using harmonized EHR data, they found that a shallow neural network using random oversampling utilizing the most common 200 EHR features, including age and sex, had an AUC of 0.80. Harmonized data means that the results can be applied to any EHR however, a simple unregularized logistic regression model of known risk factors gave an AUC of 0.79, arguing that the ML model was not substantially better than simpler models based on AF risk factors. [52]. Hill and colleagues explored neural networks for AF risk prediction in primary care practice as compared to already existing models such as CHARGE-AF, a score developed to predict incident AF in three American cohorts and validated in two European cohorts. Analysis of almost 3 million individuals identified time-varying neural networks as the optimal method of screening with an AUC of 0.827 as compared to 0.725 for CHARGE-AF, with a number needed to screen reduction by 31%, from 13 to 9 [53].

HRV is another promising variable in the detection of arrhythmias. In a study published by Chesnokov on the role of HRV in detecting PAF using AI, the artificial neural network developed was able to detect PAF in 13 patients (62 ± 21 min in advance) from non-PAF HRV [54]. A recent study used an ML approach using combined feature vector coupled with expert classification of HRV signal to detect PAF. The performance of this algorithm has shown itself to be superior to previously developed methods with a sensitivity of 100% and a specificity of 95.5% [55].

Sudden Cardiac Death

Sudden cardiac death (SCD) is the leading cause of natural death in the United States and accounts for 325,000 deaths annually and half of heart disease deaths [56]. In North America and Europe, the annual incidence of SCD ranges between 50 and 100 per 100,000 in the general population [57]. The most common cause of SCD in adults above the age of 30 is ASCVD followed by left ventricular hypertrophy. Ventricular fibrillation appears to be causing the majority of deaths [58] and its outcomes are catastrophic in the absence of early cardiopulmonary resuscitation and defibrillation. Developing methods to predict SCD events well before they occur [59] can potentially prevent some of these events or enhance survival post-arrest through rapid intervention.

Shen and colleagues created a personal cardiac homecare system by sensing the Lead-I ECG signal and trying to predict SCD events. A wavelet analysis was applied to detect SCD and the overall performance was 87.5%. They also implemented a least mean square (LMS), decision based on neural network (DBNN), and back propagation neural network with prediction rates of 67.4%, 58.1%, and 55.8% respectively [58]. To follow up on the results, Ebrahimzadeh and colleagues extracted linear, time frequency and non-linear features from HRV signals to predict SCD. When comparing it to Shen et. al's results, the predictive accuracy increased from 67.4 to 98.7% [60]. It was clear that non-linear and time frequency methods produced more accurate results. Ebrahimzadeh et al. also investigated ECG patterns up to 4 minutes before the onset of SCD. They concluded that the 2-min pre-event interval can be used to distinguish between a normal ECG and one that is prone to SCD, when every minute counts.

Polygenic Risk Scores in the Era of Machine Learning

The most widely used model for polygenic risk scores was based on linkage disequilibrium (LD) pruning of a large number of single nucleotide polymorphisms (SNPs) [61]. A study published by Abraham and colleagues showed that a polygenic risk score incorporating 49,310 variants had a discrimination ability similar to the Framingham risk score for the prediction of CAD [62]. Another study by Khera and colleagues studied genome-wide polygenic scores for common diseases; taking CAD as an example, they developed a polygenic predictor from 184,305 participants and tested their ability to predict CAD based on the UK study biobank. Their predictors had AUCs between 0.79 and 0.81 with the best score including more than 6.6 million variants. Since ML excels at analyzing large datasets, it is being explored for its application to polygenic risk scores [63].

Paré and colleagues studied a novel heuristic based on ML techniques. The group proposed to leverage the large number of SNPs and the available summary from genome wide association studies to standardize the weights of SNPs contributing to the polygenic risk score for several variables and risk factors, and then adjust for LD rather than using the conventional pruning method [64]. Their heuristic, gradient boosted and LD adjusted (GraBLD) model, used 1.98 million SNPs and yielded a prediction R^2 of 0.239 and 0.082 for height and BMI respectively, which explains 46.9 and 32.7% of the overall polygenic variance. For diabetes status, the AUC was 0.602 using the UK biobank study. GraBLD outperformed previous polygenic risk scores for prediction of height and BMI, and was noninferior to LD prediction method for diabetes [64]. Polygenic risk methods are very promising in the field of cardiovascular prevention as they allow the clinician to assess for the disease early in childhood, well before the discriminative capacity of common risk scores kick in.

A Dynamic Approach to Prevention

Beneath the dynamic approach to risk management and prediction is the concept of "initial conditions" which sets the path for changing system performances [65]. The concept represents the existing state of an organization prior to the occurrence of any hazardous events. With the distinctive sets of initial conditions, a scheme is involved in a continuous learning process that reflects a response to the initial risk and sets the upcoming state of operation [66]. To help us understand this in relation to medicine, Paltrinieri and colleagues coined the term Dynamic Risk Management Framework (DRMF), which focuses on continuous systematization of information depending on new risk evidence. The whole point of this framework is that it allows the incorporation of new input as well as continuous monitoring [67]. For example, if an individual drastically changes their diet to an unhealthy one, or starts smoking, there will be risk recalculation based on the change, allowing the process to be a continuum rather than a single snapshot. The dynamic approach to risk assessment and prevention allows for the implementation of not only primary prevention, but primordial prevention [68]. In the upcoming era of remote patient care, digital health trends such as smartphones, smart wearables and remote monitoring devices will generate a plethora of daily and real-world lifestyle and biometric data that will usher a new age of continuous risk assessment and real-time intervention. This will become the future of cardiovascular risk assessment and primary prevention.

Limitations and Future Directions

As evident from our previous discussions, the use of AI and ML in medicine and cardiology in particular, is promising. However, their use is not without challenges. The training phase is critical to develop accurate ML models, and this requires large amounts of data, good bioinformatics analytical skills and an adequate reference standard [69]. DL in particular requires a vast amount of data, which should be sufficiently labeled [8]. ML functions on the principle of "garbage in, garbage out" and inadequate data can be much more detrimental than no data. Without the availability of sufficient quality and quantity of training data, classifiers may pick up unhelpful patterns or "noise", limiting their real-life clinical applications. The first challenge comes with finding patients who are willing to share their data. While efforts are made to de-identify medical data, the risk of reidentifying the patients exist posing a risk to patient privacy [70]. Secondly, in supervised learning models, the data must be annotated by trained physicians; this can be time consuming and expensive. Moreover, these annotations may be subject to bias, which could easily get incorporated into ML models [8]. Tackling this requires careful data sampling, and efforts from the creators of the models to limit personal bias from the input data. Bias can also occur at the level of sampling, if the distribution of the training data differs from the actual setting in which the ML model will be applied [8]. Overfitting can also occur when the algorithm is excessively tuned to the training sample [69]. In this case, while the model makes very accurate predictions on its training set, its generalizability becomes limited. This can be avoided by including more data or subtly modifying the training set. Considering the pace of advancements in healthcare, ML algorithms may need to be updated frequently.

In addition to algorithm design, there are other challenges with the application of ML to health systems. Healthcare has several stakeholders, some of whom may have competing interests [8]. To successfully utilize ML in medicine, all parties must be on board. There may be resistance from healthcare professionals due to fears of being replaced, or concern over the "black box" nature of ML [8]. The decision-making processes of many ML algorithms, particularly unsupervised algorithms, are poorly understood in totality. This makes it difficult for clinicians to trust data interpretation and identify any incorrect recommendations. Patients too may want to know the reasons behind these results. As ML finds its way into clinical practice, the issue of liability should be discussed—who would be at fault if a patient is harmed due to a failure of an ML algorithm?

Development of ML techniques and their validation in cardiology is ongoing, so many of these challenges are being addressed. Efforts are underway to make integrated and curated data sets to enable ML efficacy [8]. For example, the AHA established the Precision Medicine Platform to make data easily available for researchers and improve the ease of searching across data sets [71]. Future ML-based classifier systems can be made more interpretable to increase the trust of patients and clinicians. AI can assist clinicians at every step of patient care, but cannot replace them. Rather than feel threatened by AI, clinicians should embrace it as a means for improving health care. With the advent of personalized medicine, the interest in using AI and ML in cardiology will only increase. Wearables and mobile devices are rising in popularity, and the cost of genome sequencing is decreasing, both bringing with them a plethora of available data [8]. Our community of cardiovascular practitioners should begin to get acquainted with AI and ML-based applications in cardiovascular medicine that can support their daily clinical practices.

Disclosures MBE is a co-founder of EMBER Medical, a telemedicine company.

References

1. Vakil R, et al. The future of preventive cardiology training. Am Coll Cardiol. 1(8), 201(13). www.acc.org/latest-in-cardiology/articles/2019/10/10/23/20/the-future-of-preventive-cardiology-training.
2. Shapiro, MD, et al. Preventive cardiology as a subspecialty of cardiovascular medicine: JACC Council perspectives. J Am Coll Cardiol. 2019;74(15):1926–42.
3. National Heart, Lung, and Blood Institute. Atherosclerosis Risk in Communities Study (ARIC). Operat Man. 2017;4.
4. Bild DE, et al. Multi-ethnic study of atherosclerosis: objectives and design. Am J Epidemiol. 2002;156(9):871–81.
5. Russell SJ, Norvig P. Artificial intelligence: a modern approach. Malaysia; 2016.
6. Cuocolo R, Ugga L. Imaging applications of artificial intelligence. Health Manage J. 2018;18:484–7.
7. Bishop CM. Pattern recognition and machine learning. Springer; 2006.
8. Sevakula RK, et al. State-of-the-art machine learning techniques aiming to improve patient outcomes pertaining to the cardiovascular system. J Am Heart Assoc. 2020;9(4). https://doi.org/10.1161/jaha.119.013924.
9. Rouse M. What is supervised learning? SearchEnterpriseAI, TechTarget, 10 Sept. 2019. searchenterpriseai.techtarget.com/definition/supervised-learning.
10. Heaton J. Ian Goodfellow, Yoshua Bengio, and Aaron Courville: Deep learning. Genet Prog Evol Mach. 2017;19(1–2):305–7. https://doi.org/10.1007/s10710-017-9314-z.
11. Wang J, Yang X, Cai H, Tan W, Jin C, Li L. Discrimination of breast cancer with microcalcifications on mammography by deep learning. Sci Rep. 2016;6:27327.
12. Lavecchia A. Machine-learning approaches in drug discovery: methods and applications. Drug Discov Today. 2015;20(3):318–31. https://doi.org/10.1016/j.drudis.2014.10.012.
13. Cuocolo R, et al. Current applications of Big Data and machine learning in cardiology. J Geriatr Cardiol. 2019;16(8):601–7.
14. Virani SS, et al."Heart disease and stroke statistics—2020 update: a report fromthe American Heart Association. Circulation. 2020:E139–596.
15. Perez MV, et al. Large-scale assessment of a smartwatch to identify atrial fibrillation. N E J Med. 2019;381(20):1909–17.
16. Ridker PM, Cook NR. Statins: new American guidelines for prevention of cardiovascular disease. Lancet. 2013;382:1762–5.
17. Muntner P, Colantonio LD, Cushman M, Goff DC, Howard G, Howard VJ, Kissela B, Levitan EB, Lloyd-Jones DM, Safford MM. Validation of the atherosclerotic cardiovascular disease pooled cohort risk equations. JAMA. 2014;311:1406–15.
18. Bild DE, Bluemke DA, Burke GL, Detrano R, Diez Roux AV, Folsom AR, Greenland P, Jacob DR Jr, Kronmal R, Liu K, Nelson JC, O'Leary D, Saad MF, Shea S, Szklo M, Tracy RP. Multi-ethnic study of atherosclerosis: objectives and design. Am J Epidemiol. 2002;156:871–81.
19. Kakadiaris IA, et al. Machine learning outperforms ACC/AHA CVD risk calculator in MESA. J Am Heart Assoc. 2018;7(22). https://doi.org/10.1161/jaha.118.009476.
20. Ambale-Venkatesh B, et al. Cardiovascular event prediction by machine learning. Circ Rese. 2017;121(9):1092–101. https://doi.org/10.1161/circresaha.117.311312.
21. Al'Aref SJ, et al. Machine learning of clinical variables and coronary artery calcium scoring for the prediction of obstructive coronary artery disease on coronary computed tomography angiography: analysis from the CONFIRM registry. Eur Heart J. 2019. https://doi.org/10.1093/eurheartj/ehz565.

22. Han D, et al. Machine learning framework to identify individuals at risk of rapid progression of coronary atherosclerosis: from the PARADIGM registry. J Am Heart Assoc. 2020;9(5). https://doi.org/10.1161/jaha.119.013958.

23. Oikonomou EK, et al. A novel machine learning-derived radiotranscriptomic signature of perivascular fat improves cardiac risk prediction using coronary CT angiography. Eur Heart J. 2019;40(43):3529–43. https://doi.org/10.1093/eurheartj/ehz592.

24. Antonopoulos AS, et al. Detecting human coronary inflammation by imaging perivascular fat. Sci Translat Med. 2017;9(398). https://doi.org/10.1126/scitranslmed.aal2658.

25. Oikonomou EK, et al. Non-invasive detection of coronary inflammation using computed tomography and prediction of residual cardiovascular risk (the CRISP CT study): a post-hoc analysis of prospective outcome data. The Lancet. 2018:392(10151):929–39. https://doi.org/10.1016/s0140-6736(18)31114-0.

26. Paré G, et al. A machine-learning heuristic to improve gene score prediction of polygenic traits. Sci Rep. 2017;7(1). https://doi.org/10.1038/s41598-017-13056-1.

27. Okser S, et al. Genetic variants and their interactions in the prediction of increased pre-clinical carotid atherosclerosis: the cardiovascular risk in young Finns study. PLoS Genet. 2010;6(9). https://doi.org/10.1371/journal.pgen.1001146.

28. Poplin R, et al. Prediction of cardiovascular risk factors from retinal fundus photographs via deep learning. Nat Biomed Eng. 2018;2(3):158–64. https://doi.org/10.1038/s41551-018-0195-0.

29. Wang J, et al. Detecting cardiovascular disease from mammograms with deep learning. IEEE Trans Med Imag. 2017;36(5):1172–81. https://doi.org/10.1109/tmi.2017.2655486.

30. Iribarren C, et al. Breast vascular calcification and risk of coronary heart disease, stroke, and heart failure. J Womens Health. 2004:13(4):381–9. https://doi.org/10.1089/15409990 4323087060.

31. Virani SS, et al. Heart disease and stroke statistics—2020 update: a report from the American Heart Association. Circulation. 2020;141(2). https://doi.org/10.1161/cir.0000000000000757.

32. Melillo P, Fusco R, Sansone M, et al. Discrimination power of long-term heart rate variability measures for chronic heart failure detection. Med Biol Eng Comput. 2011;49:67–74. https://doi.org/10.1007/s11517-010-0728-5.

33. Asyali MH. Discrimination power of long-term heart rate variability measures. In: Proceedings of the 25th annual international conference of the IEEE engineering in medicine and biology society (IEEE Cat. No. 03CH37439), vol. 1. IEEE; 2003.

34. İşler Y, Mehmet K. Combining classical HRV indices with wavelet entropy measures improves to performance in diagnosing congestive heart failure. Comput Biol Med. 2007;37 (10):1502–10.

35. Pecchia L, et al. Discrimination power of short-term heart rate variability measures for CHF assessment. IEEE Trans Inf Technol Biomed. 2010;15(1):40–6.

36. Liu G, et al. A new approach to detect congestive heart failure using short-term heart rate variability measures. PloS One. 2014;9(4).

37. Aljaaf AJ, et al. Predicting the likelihood of heart failure with a multi level risk assessment using decision tree. In: 2015 third international conference on technological advances in electrical, electronics and computer engineering (TAEECE). IEEE; 2015.

38. Yang G, et al. A heart failure diagnosis model based on support vector machine. In: 2010 3rd international conference on biomedical engineering and informatics, vol. 3. IEEE; 2010.

39. Zheng Y, et al. Computer-assisted diagnosis for chronic heart failure by the analysis of their cardiac reserve and heart sound characteristics. Comput Methods Prog Biomed. 2015;122 (3):372–83.

40. Choi E, et al. Using recurrent neural network models for early detection of heart failure onset. J Am Med Inf Assoc. 2017;24(2):361–70.

41. Lindholm D, et al. Bioimpedance and new-onset heart failure: a longitudinal study of >500 000 individuals from the general population. J Am Heart Assoc. 2018 7(13):e008970.

42. Go, AS, et al. Prevalence of diagnosed atrial fibrillation in adults: national implications for rhythm management and stroke prevention: the AnTicoagulation and Risk Factors in Atrial Fibrillation (ATRIA) Study. JAMA. 2001;285(18):2370–5.

43. Kannel, WB, et al. Prevalence, incidence, prognosis, and predisposing conditions for atrial fibrillation: population-based estimates. Am J Cardiol. 1998;82(7):2 N–9 N.

44. Patel, AM, et al. Treatment of underlying atrial fibrillation: paced rhythm obscures recognition. J Am Coll Cardiol. 2000;36(3):784–7.

45. Miller, PSJ, Andersson FL, Kalra L. Are cost benefits of anticoagulation for stroke prevention in atrial fibrillation underestimated? Stroke. 2005;36(2):360–6.

46. Forslund T, et al. Improved stroke prevention in atrial fibrillation after the introduction of non–vitamin K antagonist oral anticoagulants: the stockholm experience. Stroke. 2018;49 (9):2122–8.

47. Markides V, Schilling RJ. Atrial fibrillation: classification, pathophysiology, mechanisms and drug treatment. Heart. 2003;89(8):939–43.

48. Sanna T, et al. Cryptogenic stroke and underlying atrial fibrillation. N Engl J Med. 2014;370 (26):2478–86.

49. Attia ZI, et al. An artificial intelligence-enabled ECG algorithm for the identification of patients with atrial fibrillation during sinus rhythm: a retrospective analysis of outcome prediction. The Lancet. 2019;394(10201):861–7.

50. Bhalla V, et al. Diagnostic ability of B-type natriuretic peptide and impedance cardiography: testing to identify left ventricular dysfunction in hypertensive patients. Am J Hypertens. 2005;18(S2):73S–81S.

51. Wu J-T, et al. CHADS2 and CHA2DS2-VASc scores predict the risk of ischemic stroke outcome in patients with interatrial block without atrial fibrillation. J Atheroscler Thrombos. 2016:34900.

52. Tiwari P, et al. Assessment of a machine learning model applied to harmonized electronic health record data for the prediction of incident atrial fibrillation. JAMA Netw Open. 2020;3 (1):e1919396–e1919396.

53. Hill NR, et al. Predicting atrial fibrillation in primary care using machine learning. PloS One. 2019;14(11).

54. Chesnokov YV. Complexity and spectral analysis of the heart rate variability dynamics for distant prediction of paroxysmal atrial fibrillation with artificial intelligence methods. Artif Intell Med. 2008;43(2):151–65.

55. Ebrahimzadeh E, et al. Prediction of paroxysmal Atrial Fibrillation: A machine learning based approach using combined feature vector and mixture of expert classification on HRV signal. Comput Methods Prog Biomed. 2018;165:53–67.

56. "Sudden Cardiac Death (SCD): Symptoms, Causes." Cleveland Clinic, my.clevelandclinic. org/health/diseases/17522-sudden-cardiac-death-sudden-cardiac-arrest.

57. Chugh SS, et al. Current burden of sudden cardiac death: multiple source surveillance versus retrospective death certificate-based review in a large US community. J Am Coll Cardiol. 2004;44(6):1268–75.

58. Shen T-W, et al. Detection and prediction of sudden cardiac death (SCD) for personal healthcare. In: 2007 29th annual international conference of the IEEE engineering in medicine and biology society. IEEE; 2007.

59. Ichimaru Y, Kodama Y, Yanaga T. Circadian changes of heart rate variability. In: Proceedings. Computers in cardiology 1988. IEEE; 1988.

60. Ebrahimzadeh E, Pooyan M, Bijar A. A novel approach to predict sudden cardiac death (SCD) using nonlinear and time-frequency analyses from HRV signals. PloS One. 2014;9(2).

61. International Schizophrenia Consortium. Common polygenic variation contributes to risk of schizophrenia and bipolar disorder. Nature. 2009;460(7256):748.

62. Abraham G, et al. Genomic prediction of coronary heart disease. Eur Heart J. 2016;37 (43):3267–78.

63. Khera AV, et al. Genome-wide polygenic scores for common diseases identify individuals with risk equivalent to monogenic mutations. Nat Genet. 2018;50(9):1219–24.

64. Pare G, Mao S, Deng WQ. A machine-learning heuristic to improve gene score prediction of polygenic traits. Sci Rep. 2017;7(1):1–11.
65. Kauffman SA. The origins of order: self-organization and selection in evolution. USA: Oxford University Press; 1993.
66. Paltrinieri N, Louise C, Genserik R. Learning about risk: machine learning for risk assessment. Saf Sci. 2019;118:475–86.
67. Paltrinieri N, et al. Dynamic approach to risk management: Application to the Hoeganaes metal dust accidents. Process Saf Environ Prot. 2014;92(6):669–79.
68. Vaduganathan M, Venkataramani AS, Bhatt DL. Moving toward global primordial prevention in cardiovascular disease: the heart of the matter. 2015:1535–7.
69. Cuocolo R, et al. Current applications of Big Data and machine learning in cardiology. J Geriatr Cardiol. 2019;16(8):601–7. PubMed. www.ncbi.nlm.nih.gov/pmc/articles/PMC6748901/#!po=58.3333, https://doi.org/10.11909/j.issn.1671-5411.2019.08.002. Accessed 10 Apr 2020.
70. Emam KEl, et al. Evaluating the risk of re-identification of patients from hospital prescription records. Can J Hosp Pharm. 2009;62(4). https://doi.org/10.4212/cjhp.v62i4.812.
71. Kass-Hout TA, et al. American Heart Association precision medicine platform. Circulation. 2018;137(7):647–9. https://doi.org/10.1161/circulationaha.117.032041.
72. Dhall D, Kaur R, Juneja M. Machine learning: A review of the algorithms and its applications. In: Singh P, Kar A, Singh Y, Kolekar M, Tanwar S (eds) Proceedings of ICRIC 2019. Lecture Notes in Electrical Engineering, vol 597. Springer, Cham (2020). https://doi.org/10.1007/978-3-030-29407-6_5.

Novel Research Designs

Anjali Wagle, Nino Isakadze, and Seth S. Martin

Introduction

Medicine is constantly evolving. Now, more than ever, we are seeing an exponential growth of therapeutics particularly capitalizing on technological advances. Healthcare providers have found ways to provide medical care outside of the classic clinic or hospitalist visit and the techniques continue to grow. In the past few years we have seen increasing use of electronic devices for patient care, medical education, and clinical guidance. Through more accessible monitoring and reporting at both the individual and population level, mobile applications have the potential to greatly improve our diagnosis and treatment of health conditions as well as reduce the cost of health care. What is currently lacking in this new paradigm is not innovation in technology, but innovation in how technology is evaluated. The present landscape does not have research methods with the necessary rigor and efficiency to monitor the efficacy and challenges of these new interventions. Of particular importance is developing a method to evaluate technology at a rate that keeps up with the pace of creation. The aim of this chapter will be to discuss the limitations of our current techniques in evaluating mobile health (mHealth) technology as well as providing an introduction to new methods created for this purpose.

A. Wagle · N. Isakadze
Johns Hopkins University, Baltimore, USA

S. S. Martin (✉)
Digital Health Innovation Laboratory, Ciccarone Center for the Prevention of Cardiovascular Disease, Division of Cardiology, Department of Medicine, Johns Hopkins University School of Medicine, Johns Hopkins Hospital, 600 N. Wolfe St., Carnegie 568, Baltimore, MD 21287, US
e-mail: smart100@jhmi.edu

© Springer Nature Switzerland AG 2021   149
S. S. Martin (ed.), *Precision Medicine in Cardiovascular Disease Prevention*,
https://doi.org/10.1007/978-3-030-75055-8_7

History of RCTs

Randomized controlled trials have long been considered the gold standard of evidenced based medicine. The first randomized controlled trial is typically attributed to the British Medical Research Council's (MRC) evaluation of streptomycin for the treatment of tuberculosis in 1948 [1]. Prior to the MRC trial, researchers strove to evaluate therapeutic efficacy of interventions using case reports, case series, clinical reasoning, and prior experience. However, the prevailing methodology was the alternate-allocation scheme that involved treating every other patient in a research cohort. However, in the 1930s, concerns about selection bias led Dr. Bradford Hill to devise a new methodology for the MRC trial that was without the limitations of alternate-allocation trials. The MRC was one of the first trials to assign patients in a randomized fashion and to conceal patient assignments from researchers. In doing so, Dr. Hill demonstrated how to proactively address selection bias and established the importance of blinded randomized trials.

The RCT carved a place for itself in the United States particularly after World War II, when the medical community was trying to make sense of the pharmaceutical revolution that had recently occurred. Pharmaceutical companies were reluctant to spend even more resources and potentially delay approval for their drug in order to test for efficacy. The unsustainable system revealed its flaws in 1961 when a new drug, thalidomide, was prescribed to thousands of pregnant women. The subsequent years were marked by an international epidemic of stillbirths and malformed neonatal limbs, eventually traced back to the "mild sleeping pill". In response, between the 1960s and 70s, the Food and Drug Administration mandated proof of efficacy of new drug applications in the form of RCT results [2, 3]. The U.S. was closely followed by other national regulatory agencies including the Japanese government and the Council of the European Economic Community. To comply with the new regulations, the pharmaceutical industry became a leading sponsor of RCTs while medical researchers promoted RCTs as a way to make medicine more rational [4]. The RCT thus became the most vigorous representation of study designs aimed to adjudicate clinical efficacy and address research bias.

Benefits of RCTs

Over the past 50 years, RCTs have undergone development and refinement making it one of the highest levels of evidence in EBM. Qualities unique to RCTs include randomization, blinding, and placebo control, making RCTs the reference standard for driving practice.

All study designs aim to yield objective data with bias minimized. A major way that RCTs provide this is by randomization, where participants are randomly assigned to different intervention or placebo conditions. Selection bias occurs when there are nonrandom factors that can influence enrollment in either arm of a study.

Randomization protects against selection bias because there cannot be a priori knowledge of group assignment with randomization techniques. This is also known as allocation concealment, which keeps clinicians and participants unaware of the participants' assignments. Pharmaceutical trials are well suited to allocation concealment since a matching placebo can be manufactured. Failure of allocation concealment leads to exaggerated positive and negative estimates of treatment effects [5].

In observational studies, causal interpretation is more limited than in RCTs because of the numerous confounding variables that are not adjusted for or incompletely adjusted for. Randomization provides a fundamental tool for researchers to attempt to minimize confounding in treatment assignment by producing separate groups in which influencing prognostic factors and other baseline covariates, known and unknown, can have symmetry. Randomization can be as simple as flipping a coin, however, this can lead to inter-group chance imbalances. This imbalance of baseline characteristics can influence comparison between treatment and control groups and introduce confounding factors. Various techniques have thus been developed to address this issue including different ways to randomize participants [6–8]. Examples include simple, block, stratified and covariate adaptive randomizations. Each randomization method is used in specific situations as each method has a particular set of advantages and disadvantages [9]. As a result of randomization, baseline characteristics are often well balanced between the comparative groups as classically presented in the first table of RCT manuscripts [10].

RCTs have contributed to developing successful treatments for cardiovascular health. Some of the first, large randomized controlled trials in cardiology include the International Study of Infarct Survival (ISIS) and Gruppo Italiano per lo Studio della Streptochinasi nell'Infarto Miocardico (GISSI) series of trials which concluded that beta blockers, aspirin, thrombotic therapy, and angiotensin converting enzyme inhibitors are beneficial in patients with ischemia [11, 12]. Key aspects of these trials were the large trial size and simplicity in design that made these studies practical and cost effective.

Limitations of RCTs

While RCTs have become the standard in research and cardiology guidelines, the medical community still frequently utilizes "lower-tiers" of evidence to inform practice. This is largely because we lack RCTs for many of the common clinical questions that face patients and clinicians. Furthermore, other methods may be well suited to answer the clinical question such as questions about diagnostic performance or natural history.

In order for data gleaned from an RCT to become clinically useful, it must minimize the possibility of bias and have a result that is clearly applicable to a defined group of people, also known as internal and external validity, respectfully. While there have been many methods to optimize internal validity, lack of external validity is one of the most frequent criticisms by clinicians of RCTs [13–17].

External validity can be compromised by the eligibility criteria, subject recruitment, or diagnosis definition. Many RCTs exclude pregnant women and the elderly [18]. Other RCTs exclude patients with comorbidities that are highly prevalent in the general population, also making the trial less generalizable.

Such assessments from trial data must reconcile the difference of benefits and harms ascertained at a group level with how that translates to individual patient care. Usually, published trials include baseline characteristics of their patient population from which clinicians can assess external validity by comparing with their patient. However, comparing baseline clinical characteristics have proven misleading because patients may differ from the trial population in seemingly inconsequential attributes that later are deemed to have a major effect on the end result.

Another limitation many RCTs face is the increasingly high cost and time demands required to complete a trial. Given the complexity, RCTs often take years to plan, implement, and analyze, which can reduce their utility in some instances. In urgent public health crises, for example, clinicians initially rely on case studies and anecdotal information to guide treatment as RCTs are developed and conducted. Additionally, in rapidly evolving specialties, RCTs may have outdated therapies by the time they publish.

There are countless other examples of the limitations of RCTs including the difficulty of identifying rare but serious adverse effects and limited ability to detect individualized effect of a treatment [4]. Judging if an RCT is applicable for an individual patient falls on the shoulders of clinicians and in areas of large information gaps new ways to obtain clinical data on interventions have been recently gaining favor [19].

In this chapter, we describe how technology is being leveraged to better understand and improve health. Additionally, we aim to describe new ways to analyze these digital health interventions, illustrate key limitations of each method, and suggest when they are appropriate (Table 1).

Micro-randomized Trials

Summary of the Design

In the past, interventions largely took the form of medications or in-office procedures. However, with the advent of largely ubiquitous mobile phone ownership there has been an interest in leveraging personalized technology to understand and improve health. One recent development in mHealth intervention includes just-in-time adaptive interventions, or JITAIs. For JITAIs, the intervention can be as simple as sending a motivational message through text messaging. These interventions can be sent multiple times per day depending on the type of intervention. While there have been numerous JITAIs created, data have largely lagged behind as the research interventions are created faster than current research methods can prove their efficacy.

Table 1 Advantages and disadvantages of innovative research designs to drive precision medicine forward

Name of design	Example	Advantages	Disadvantages
MRT	HeartSteps physical activity study	• Multiple randomizations allow for causal inferences to be made • Optimized for behavioral interventions • Can better identify which component of the intervention is effective	• The method for MRTs are not ideal for optional interventions • Not suited for situations and interventions that are rare
N-of-1	N-of-1 (single-patient) trials for statin related myalgias	• Evaluate short-term outcomes Appropriate to determine effect of intervention on individual basis rather than the population level • Able to focus on patient reported symptoms	• Challenge with generalizing the results • Time-intensive for staff to conduct the study for few individuals
Patient centered participatory research	Diabetes Networking Tool	• Involves the target audience of the application to make it more user friendly and provides better understanding of the needs for the application • Transparency of the limitations with users	• Members of the team will have variable expertise with mHealth tools • Incorporating ideas from a wide variety of participants may increase the amount of time and money required
Site-less trials	Apple Heart Study	• Decreases the time and cost of running a clinical trial • Increases patient participation by decreasing barriers of traveling • Allows increased participation from patients who live in remote areas	• Inappropriate to study medications with uncertain safety profiles • Not as beneficial of a design in trials that involve medical imaging or medically administered medications
Stepped Wedged Trial	High-Sensitivity Cardiac Troponin and the Universal Definition of Myocardial Infarction	• Allows participants to trial both the intervention and the control	• May prolong trial timeline as all participants will need to trial the intervention and control

The micro-randomized trial (MRT) is an example of an alternative to traditional parallel-group randomized controlled trials [20, 21]. In this method, the treatments under study and a control are randomly assigned to an individual at each decision point throughout the entirety of the study (Fig. 1). The treatment recommendations can include engagement and/or therapeutic treatment that rely on self-reported or gathered user-specific information to provide personalized recommendations. The decision point is a specific time when the study intervention might be efficacious for the participant, which is initially based on theory, the individual's past behavior, and current context. The decision points can be location, time, or trigger based depending on the type of study. For example, if a study was interested in the effect of a message encouraging the individual to take his or her medication at a specific time, the decision point would be the medication time. An example of a location guided decision point would be if a study was interested in the effect of a message discouraging alcohol use, then every time the participant was within 5 feet of an alcohol store the message would be sent.

A key feature of the MRT is defining proximal and distal outcomes. Proximal outcomes are similar to primary outcomes of an RCT, meaning the goal behavioral change that occurs immediately after an intervention is deployed. In the first example above, a proximal outcome could be to measure the number of days in a week that a participant was adherent to his or her medication. Proximal outcomes are often seen as building blocks to the distal outcome. The distal outcomes are often the amalgamation of the proximal outcomes at each decision point over a certain period of time. The distal outcome in this example could be the number of heart failure exacerbations a patient has in 6 months if the medications targeted for adherence include heart failure medications.

Another group of effects MRTs can study are lagged effects. Lagged effects are changes in behavior that are due to the intervention but are outside the window period of a proximal effect. These effects are important to determine decision point characteristics. If the proximal outcomes show low medication adherence, lagged effects may still be present. In particular, a delayed but sustained increase in medication adherence suggests that the intervention had some effect, but additionally that number or timing of the intervention can be changed perhaps to elicit an effect more proximally.

Pros and Cons

Micro-randomized trials (MRTs) have been able to optimize JITAI's for two main reasons. First, because the interventions are repeatedly randomized, MRTs allow researchers to understand how the causal effects vary over time, in different conditions, and with individual factors. JITAI's have largely used multicomponent behavioral interventions such as targeting cardiovascular disease with messaging that encourages adherence with the prescribed medication, exercise, and diet regimen. Previously, such trials were assessed using an RCT to determine if these

A. Micro-randomized trial design:

	Validation phase		Decision Point 1	Decision Point 2	Decision Point 3	Decision Point 4	Decision Point 5	Decision Point 6	Decision Point 7	Decision Point 8
Participant 1	Control		Control	Intervention A	Intervention B	Intervention B	Intervention A	Control	Intervention B	Intervention A
Participant 2	Control		Intervention A	Control	Intervention A	Intervention B	Intervention B	Intervention B	Intervention A	Control
Participant 3	Control		Intervention A	Intervention A	Intervention B	Control	Intervention A	Control	Intervention B	Intervention B

B. N-of-1 trial design:

	Validation phase		Decision Point 1	Decision Point 2	Decision Point 3	Decision Point 4	Decision Point 5	Decision Point 6
Participant 1	Control		Intervention A	Control	Intervention A	Control	Intervention A	Control

C. Patient-centered participatory research design:

D. Site-less trial design:

E. Stepped-wedge trial design:

	Validation phase		Decision Point 1	Decision Point 2	Decision Point 3
Participant 1	Control		Intervention A	Intervention A	Intervention A
Participant 2	Control		Control	Intervention A	Intervention A
Participant 3	Control		Control	Control	Intervention A

Fig. 1 Visualizations of innovative research designs to drive precision medicine forward: micro-randomized, n-of-1, stepped wedge, site-less, and patient participatory designs. Section A illustrates an example of a MRT. All participants initially are monitored with the control during the validation phase. With each decision point, the participant may be randomized to any of the interventions or the control. Section B describes how during n-of-1 trials there is one participant who is monitored on a control and then may cross-over back and forth between and intervention and control, possibly with a washout. Section C, patient-centered participatory design, is where the end-user or patient is engaged in all steps of the product development process. Section D gives an example of a site-less design where the entire study is conducted without person-to-person interaction. Section E shows the Stepped-Wedge trial design which gradually integrates the intervention until all participants are in the intervention arm by the end of the trial

interventions had an effect on the behavior of interest. However, RCTs were optimized to evaluate single-component interventions and when they are applied to multi-component interventions there are some challenges in the protocol. The RCT was not designed to investigate the particular components of the intervention (when is it efficacious, what contextual or psychosocial factors influenced the efficacy, or what particular components of the intervention were effective) only the intervention as a whole. However, to optimize JITAI's it is crucial to first understand what impacts the intervention's target end points.

Another downstream effect of repeatedly randomizing interventions for the same participant is that this allows researchers to understand time-varying effects of an intervention. Through MRT's researchers can study how a participant responds to JITAI over time and in differing psychosocial and contextual conditions. Additionally, this type of randomization, because it is done at every decision point, can randomize a participant hundreds of times in the course of a month, depending on the trial. Analysis can be done not only in the classical manner of comparing participants in the intervention group and the placebo group, but also since each individual is randomized multiple times to a different or no intervention, analysis can be done on the contrasts in outcomes for one person. This allows MRT studies to require a fewer total number of participants than classic research methods would dictate. Randomization of this magnitude makes MRTs highly efficient research methods which is why they are helpful to keep up with the fast-paced innovation of JITAIs.

There are a few limitations of MRTs. First, these trials are only available to test interventions that send reminders or prompts to individuals rather than interventions that the participants can access optionally. Second, given that individuals are receiving these interventions likely in the context of interruptions, MRTs are best suited to interventions for which the proximal outcomes are easily tracked either passively or through brief self-report given the repeated number of times an individual will have an intervention. Lastly, these trials are well suited for testing interventions that occur often.

MRT Example

An example of an MRT study and JITAI is the HeartSteps physical activity study, a JITAI developed to help individuals increase their physical activity, primarily through walking [20]. In this study, through sensors and user surveys, information about the users' context such as location, time of day, day of week, and weather is gathered to customize every suggestion for how users can be active in their current environment. The HeartSteps team conducted an MRT to assess the efficacy of these activity suggestions to evaluate whether the participants had a proximal increase in physical activity following the interventions and if the effect varied over time.

HeartSteps would only deliver activity suggestions to participants if they were deemed available for treatment. The users were considered "unavailable" while driving, if the participant was already currently walking or running, if the participant recently finished an activity on the last 90s, and if their phone was offline.

For each decision point that a user was considered available, the HeartSteps server micro-randomized the delivery of the activity suggestion. Each suggestion was treated as independent from prior suggestions. The possible suggestions included walking, anti-sedentary, and no suggestions. The anti-sedentary suggestions were included as an engagement strategy to add variety with activities such as stretching, jumping jacks, etc. The 37 participants generated 8,274 person-decision points over the course of the 6-week study period.

The study showed that each suggestion results in an additional 35 steps totaling around 100 steps over the course of the day. The MRT found that the walking suggestions performed better than anti-sedentary suggestions. Additionally, due to the MRT design, the study was able to demonstrate that tailoring suggestions to user context influenced the efficacy of the suggestions and that the potency of suggestions diminished over time likely due to habituation.

Other examples of current MRTs include Sense2Stop, investigating JITAIs using sensor-based assessments of stress to aid in smoking cessation. Another is the BaraFIT MRT aiming to promote weight maintenance status post bariatric surgery by using the JITAI approach in text messages encouraging physical activity and improved diets.

N-of-1

Summary of the Design

For every medical decision, clinicians are tasked with applying results from guidelines, RCTs, and other published data to their patient. As mentioned in the first section, this can be challenging for many reasons including heterogeneous effects in study populations and external validity concerns of the trials.

Additionally, there is growing interest in understanding the individual variables of a person that impact treatment effectiveness and adverse effects. This field of medicine has had particular success in oncological research where many cancer therapeutic profiles are influenced by genomic profiles causing the US FDA to require genetic profiling prior to administering certain treatments [22]. Similarly, in other fields of medicine there have been attempts to estimate individual treatment effects (ITE) indirectly, most notably through subgroup analyses. However, this method has been criticized due to problems associated with multiple testing causing an increase in the false-positive rate.

Reconciling the growing interest in precision medicine and the need for evidence based practicing has led to a plethora of new methods including the N-of-1 trial.

N-of-1 trials are single-patient trials of treatment effectiveness and safety. The design of an "n-of-1" trial is based on conventional research methods that are already in wide-use for population-based trials. They model RCTs in design in that they are double blind and randomized in order to minimize bias. However, the key difference between n-of-1 trials and conventional trials is that n-of-1 trials revolve around one individual, which allows researchers to ascertain benefit and safety on an individual level to allow for objective determination of the optimal therapy for an individual patient.

The main method of n-of-1 trials lies in the simple crossover design in which the administration order of two compounds, either two treatments or one treatment and one placebo, is randomized across multiple periods for one individual (Fig. 1). This type of design is commonly referred to as "ABAB" design with "A" referring to an intervention and "B" referring to a placebo or second intervention. The timing of each intervention period would be based on the characteristics of the outcome and therapy with particular thought given to minimizing carryover effects. Repeated number of periods of "ABAB" can be performed to reduce confounding variables.

Pros and Cons

A key advantage found in n-of-1 trials is the ability to evaluate causality at the individual level for short-term outcomes. Whereas traditional RCTs are unable to detect uncommon but troublesome adverse drug effects, and unable to assess if they are causal in nature in individuals who experience them, the n-of-1 trial can be applied in this setting. An important part of planning an n-of-1 trial is defining the treatment target to select symptoms that have been particularly troublesome for the individual patient in order to capitalize on the advantage of n-of-1 trial design.

While n-of-1 trials have a long history in education and psychology, the rise of this design in clinical medicine has been slow to date for a variety of reasons [23]. For a clinician, the barriers predominantly include time and cost. In order to start a clinical n-of-1 trial with a patient the clinician must discuss their idea with the patient, see them regularly throughout the trial, and evaluate their symptoms at specific time points. With increasingly shortened clinic visits and over-booked clinicians, having a physician spend an increased amount of time conducting these meetings can be a significant burden on their clinic schedule. Other challenges with n-of-1 trials include that not all clinical conditions are optimized to be tested with an n-of-1 trial, and furthermore IRB approval and consent may be needed, and the cost of manufacturing matching placebos.

Another often noted challenge with n-of-1 trials include the lack of generalizability often makes it difficult to disseminate the data. However, while this is true, if concurrent n-of-1 trials testing the same intervention in multiple patients are conducted then a possible solution could involve meta-analyses on data generated from the individual trials [24]. An advantage of starting with an individual approach and then broadening it to the more generalizable population analysis is that each participant involved in an n-of-1 trial has an opportunity to benefit immediately from the information obtained. This is in contrast to RCTs where a patient may be on placebo during the whole study period.

Example of N-of-1 Trials

A classic n-of-1 trial focused on statin associated muscle symptom in 8 patients who had high 10-year Framingham cardiovascular risk profiles [25]. Each of these patients had developed myalgia within three weeks of starting a statin, which allowed for the treatment period to be set to three weeks for each intervention arm: placebo and statin. The study design included three pairs of three weeks of active treatment and three weeks of placebo with an equivalent washout period in between to minimize carryover effects. The statin used for treatment was the same type of statin and dose that the patient had previously ascribed their myalgia to. A computer-generated algorithm randomly determined the order of the treatment or placebo during the treatment pair. The protocol maintained blinding by creating identical bottles and capsules that were compounded by the hospital pharmacy. Additionally, physicians and other staff were also blinded to the treatment sequence.

The study assessed patient symptoms using two different visual analogue scales (VAS) and the Brief Pain Inventory (BPI) short form [26]. The visual analogue scales assessed the patient's level of muscle pain as well as the intensity of a pre-determined symptom (thought to be from statin initiation) that was most bothersome to the individual patient. The symptom assessments were completed on a weekly basis during the treatment periods.

Data analysis of the patients' self-reported VAS myalgia scores, symptom specific VAS score, or BPI found no statistically significant difference in myalgia during the statin and placebo periods. Considering these results, most of the patients (5 of 8) in the study population restarted their statin therapy after the trial.

There are many advantages of using an n-of-1 trial design to assess statin associated muscle symptoms. Standard practice when a patient endorses statin-related myalgia would be to discontinue then rechallenge, lower the dose, start a different type of statin, or discontinue statin use indefinitely. With exception to the last option, many times these patients have persistent muscle symptoms that are not definitively attributable to statin use and until n-of-1 trials, there have not been systematic ways to gain further understanding of if patients should be taken off of a statin. This n-of-1 trial was able to control for biases to determine whether the myalgia was caused by statin use. Additionally, since the trial was an n-of-1 design, the researchers were also able to assess individualized symptoms that were most bothersome to the patient that was initially thought to be statin-related. By individualizing the symptom assessments, the result of the n-of-1 trial showing that the symptoms were not significantly increased during the statin periods was able to convince patients to restart their statin.

Patient Centered Participatory Research/User Centered Design

Summary of Design

A large part of precision medicine includes using mHealth tools to empower patients to take a more active role in their medical care. mHealth tools have been used to improve patient communication, access to health services, treatment adherence and chronic disease management [27–29]. However, mHealth tools have had variable attrition rates and usability problems often attributed to the method of development. The predominant culture of mHealth tool development is characterized by an expert mind-set, where the end-user takes a passive role. The converse method is a participatory mind-set which views the end-user as co-creators in the design process [30]. Many mHealth tools are constructed with marginal, if any, engagement from the end-user, which leads to disconnect in usability, effectiveness, and sustainability of the applications [31–33].

User-centered design (UCD) refers to a method of creating mHealth tools based on discussions with the ultimate end-user of the tool. This is in contrast to developing an app based off of opinions from an engineer or medical expert in the topic or large data analyses [34]. The eventual goals of such a patient-facing process are to increase patient self-sufficiency and deliver a tool that needs minimum effort to learn how to use it.

Participatory design (PD) is a subset of UCD. It is a qualitative research method, primarily used in mHealth interventions, that aims to bring in users as "co-investigators" in the design process to better align the technology with the eventual users. Whereas UCD observes how users interact with the current system and understands their thought processes behind their opinions to then later independently develop a new system, PD invites users to the development of the new system. The main principles of PD include a mutual exchange of ideas between designers and users to better understand the needs of the technology, equalization of power amongst the group, and framing of design tasks in ways that allow end-users the ability to communicate and participate in the design process [35].

Pros and Cons

The main advantages of UCD and PD is that by directly involving the target audience of the technology in the design process the team will receive a better understanding of the social, practical, and psychological factors behind the usability of a mHealth tool. Incorporating the end-users in the development process will lead to products that are more user-friendly, efficient, effective, and sustainable. Additionally, involving patients could also have a benefit of increasing their sense of ownership in the product and over their disease.

Another advantage of these methods is to be transparent about the limitations in design and functionality to users. Understanding why a function is not present could help manage expectations and result in a smoother integration of the product into the environment.

The main disadvantage precluding this type of design from most development plans is that to gather data from users takes time and money. Additionally, with many members of the team with differing expertise and experience with mHealth tools there has to be an emphasis on communicating effectively and respectfully. Lastly, including focus groups of users may create a tool that is developed to tailor to a small group of people and be less generalizable for a larger population.

Example of PD

The Diabetes Networking Tool (DNT) was created as a mHealth tool to improve health outcomes in patients with type 2 diabetes by bolstering their social support network to help meet these needs [36]. The researchers used a PD to involve a low-income, predominantly African American community with a high burden of diabetes in the developmental process of the DNT.

There were a total of four forums over a three-month period that involved various members of the community (end-users) as well as user-interface, mHealth, and public health experts. The user-interface and mHealth experts' roles were to ensure the ideas developed during these forms were feasible for the DNT. There were four forums held which centered on the users desires for functionality and user experience of the app. Each forum had a moderator, and the activities of the forum were recorded in a variety of ways.

By the end of the four forums, 29 specific functions for the DNT had emerged. In order to reduce the functional goals of the app with the hopes of increasing usability, the team distributed a survey of the potential functions to a subcommittee of technology developers, community engagement researchers, and clinicians to rank each function as low, medium, or high priority. Functions were removed from consideration due to low priority rankings, technicalities such as coding difficulties, and cost constraints, ultimately establishing a list of ten community-suggested DNT functions for inclusion in the final design. These ten functions were then grouped into four groups, each of which was the task of a different content group. The four groups included: remind, share, active, and learn and are available at the bottom of the DNT screen.

In addition to guiding the functionality of the app, the forums with community members also revealed other aspects of the app that impact usability. For example, many members of the community shared that, due to their diabetes, they have developed vision and fine-motor issues. The team used that information and created pages with larger fonts and simple gesture interactions.

Site-Less/Digital Clinical Trials

Summary of Design

Currently, the pace of clinical trials and the development of mHealth tools have been incongruent, resulting in needless halting of the development and distribution of apps aimed to help the population's health. The period of clinical testing is particularly burdensome both from a financial and timeline perspective with some estimates proposing that it takes about 10 years to bring a new entity through research and development [37]. A significant amount of the cost involves site-monitoring alone, comprising between 9 and 14% of overall expenditures [38]. Recruitment and retention of participants also pose an additional risk largely due to varying proximity of patient homes to the academic center and the inconvenience associated with multiple patient visits [39].

Research groups have developed creative means around these barriers including the site-less clinical trials. As the naming suggests, site-less clinical trials are based on patient location rather than the academic center. Many of these trials use video-conferencing, wearable sensors, and other telehealth initiatives to conduct the recruitment and/or the study period which has decreased the number of visits, time, and cost of research initiatives [40]. If 'visits' are needed they can be implemented through synchronous (same time) or asynchronous (different time) communication platforms [41]. The advent of site-less trials became popular after 2015 when the FDA solicited feedback on individual and industry experiences with the use of technology in the conduct of clinical investigation.

One of the first European remote clinic studies without a single site visit was used to assess the utility of a wireless glucometer in patients with diabetes [42]. Participants were recruited through Facebook, registered online through a cloud platform, reviewed patient information documents, and signed an online informed consent document. Study materials were delivered to the patients' houses where they connected the wireless glucometer with their personal online account. With the site-less design, compliance was shown to improve 18% and the study site estimated spending 66% less time in care coordination activities which represents a significant improvement in patient convenience and clinical efficiency [43].

Pros and Cons

Site-less clinical trials have been used to decrease the time and cost of running a clinical trial as well as increase patient participation by decreasing burden. Additionally, this method would be especially helpful in special populations such as rare diseases, patients with disabilities, patients who live in remote areas where typical studies usually require traveling long distances to participate. The virtual aspect of the trial also lends itself to home-observation of clinical symptoms, as will be discussed in the next section.

There are aspects of some clinical trials, however, that make the site-less design not appropriate. These trials include those that require medically administered medications, medications with uncertain safety profile, and trials that require regular medical imaging [44].

Example of a Site-Less Design

One of the most ubiquitous phones and watches, the Apple iPhone and Watch were recently evaluated in the Apple Heart Study to determine if an irregular pulse notification algorithm can aid in identifying atrial fibrillation [45]. Potential participants were sent a single email to Apple Watch owners inviting them to participate. The trial was able to recruit 419,297 participants in 8 months. The study app was used to verify eligibility, obtain participants' consent, provide study education, and explain the study procedures. Once the participant provided consent, the irregular pulse notification algorithm was automatically activated.

The participants were prompted from the study app to initiate occasional telemedicine visits, which were conducted by a physician. If a patient was found to have an irregular rhythm and was deemed stable, the patient would receive an ECG patch to wear for 7 days after which they were returned and read by two clinicians. 2161 patients received in irregular pulse notification and were mailed an ECG patch. 450 participants returned their ECG strip to be analyzed. The trial found a positive predictive value of 0.84 in patients who received an irregular pulse notification that was later confirmed on the ECG patch. Additionally, the trial found atrial fibrillation present in 34% of patients overall among participants who received an irregular rhythm notification. The site-less design of the Apple Heart Study allowed for widespread enrollment in only 8 months with diversity in geography, race and ethnicity.

Stepped Wedge Trial

Summary of Design

A stepped wedge trial (SWT) is a method that uses a sequential rollout of the intervention to all of the participants within the study [46]. With the SWT, all participants begin in the control group. After a pre-specified time, a set amount of participants will initiate the intervention while the remaining participants will continue with the control (Fig. 1). This will continue to happen until all participants have crossed over into the intervention arm. There are two classifications of SWT that depend on how which participants are measured within a cluster [47]. If the same participants are measured at each measurement occasion then the design is called a cohort SWT. Alternatively, if the participants measured at the measurement occasion are randomly chosen each time then it is called a cross-sectional SWT.

Pros and Cons

The SWT design is particularly useful in cases where the intervention is expected to be superior to the control. In these situations, there has been an ethical dilemma when assessing the intervention using a traditional parallel design because the intervention is being withheld from one group. In the SWT, all participants have access to the intervention at some point during the study period. Additionally, because the participants will have experienced both the intervention and the control the SWT can compare individuals to themselves and reduce unmeasured confounders.

The main disadvantage of a SWT is that it can take longer to complete the trial since the participants enter the intervention period at differing times and all participants must have the intervention. The SWT may also be difficult because there may be practical hurdles in providing all of the participants with the intervention. Additionally, a SWT is not suited to test multiple types of interventions. Lastly, blinding is particularly difficult in a SWT given that all participants would be aware of the change in protocol when they transition from the control to intervention.

Example of Stepped Wedged Trial Design

The SWT design was used to investigate the implementation of high sensitivity cardiac troponin (hs-cTnI) assays in a study by Chapman et al. [48]. The study used a validation period of 6–12 months where the results of the hs-cTn1 were concealed from the attending physician and management was driven based off of the contemporary troponin assay (cTnI). There were 10 hospitals who participated and were randomly assigned when they would advance to the intervention phase. The study used national registries to ensure follow up after hospitalization with primary outcomes being subsequent myocardial infarction or cardiovascular death within 1 year following the hospitalization. About 17% of patients were reclassified after introduction of high-sensitivity troponin, however, the incidence of subsequent MI and cardiovascular death was not changed. The SWT design allowed for analysis to be down between hospitals with different randomization outcomes as well as within one hospital using pre and post intervention data.

Summary/Conclusion

Medicine is moving towards a more individualized approach with technological advancements increasingly tailored towards specific patients. mHealth technologies have included using smart phone applications, wearable devices, and hand held devices, among others to provide real-time monitoring of physiologic measurements. This innovation has started to change the way that healthcare services are organized and delivered which has consequences for the generation of clinical evidence. The novel research designs highlighted in this chapter will drive precision medicine forward by changing the way evidence-based and individualized medicine are pursued. These methods will help move research from population-averaged effects to those directly relevant to the individual. While the RCT remains an important standard, it has its own limitations and these novel research designs have the capacity to more accurately match the research method to the clinical question. Further development and understanding of research methods to assess mHealth technologies is critical.

References

 1. Bothwell LE, Podolsky SH. The emergence of the randomized. Controlled Trial. N Engl J Med. 2016;375(6):501–4.
 2. Carpenter D, Reputation and power: organizational image and pharmaceutical regulation at the FDA. Princeton University Press; 2010.
 3. Greene JA, Podolsky SH. Reform, regulation, and pharmaceuticals—the Kefauver-Harris Amendments at 50. N Engl J Med. 2012;367(16):1481–3.
 4. Bothwell LE, et al. Assessing the gold standard-lessons from the history of RCTs. N Engl J Med. 2016;374(22):2175–81.
 5. Schulz KF, Grimes DA. Allocation concealment in randomised trials: defending against deciphering. Lancet. 2002;359(9306):614–8.
 6. Lin Y, Zhu M, Su Z. The pursuit of balance: an overview of covariate-adaptive randomization techniques in clinical trials. Contemp Clin Trials. 2015;45(Pt A):21–5.
 7. Pocock SJ, Simon R. Sequential treatment assignment with balancing for prognostic factors in the controlled clinical trial. Biometrics. 1975;31(1):103–15.
 8. Stanley K. Design of randomized controlled trials. Circulation. 2007;115(9):1164–9.
 9. Scott NW, et al. The method of minimization for allocation to clinical trials. A review. Control Clin Trials. 2002;23(6):662–74.
10. Altman DG, et al. The revised CONSORT statement for reporting randomized trials: explanation and elaboration. Ann Intern Med. 2001;134(8):663–94.
11. Randomised trial of intravenous atenolol among 16 027 cases of suspected acute myocardial infarction: ISIS-1. First International Study of Infarct Survival Collaborative Group. Lancet. 1986;2(8498):57–66.
12. Long-term effects of intravenous thrombolysis in acute myocardial infarction: final report of the GISSI study. Gruppo Italiano per lo Studio della Streptochi-nasi nell'Infarto Miocardico (GISSI). Lancet. 1987;2(8564):871–4.
13. Evans JG. Evidence-based and evidence-biased medicine. Age Ageing. 1995;24(6):461–3.
14. Naylor CD. Grey zones of clinical practice: some limits to evidence-based medicine. Lancet. 1995;345(8953):840–2.

15. Garfield FB, Garfield JM. Clinical judgment and clinical practice guidelines. Int J Technol Assess Health Care. 2000;16(4):1050–60.
16. Cabana MB, Powe NR, et al. Why don't clinicians follow clinical practice guidelines? A framework for improvement. JAMA. 1999;282:1458–65.
17. Sonis J, et al. Applicability of clinical trial results to primary care. JAMA. 1998;280 (20):1746.
18. Gurwitz JH, Col NF, Avorn J. The exclusion of the elderly and women from clinical trials in acute myocardial infarction. JAMA. 1992;268(11):1417–22.
19. Frieden TR. Evidence for health decision making—beyond randomized. Controlled Trials. N Engl J Med. 2017;377(5):465–75.
20. Liao P, et al. Sample size calculations for micro-randomized trials in mHealth. Stat Med. 2016;35(12):1944–71.
21. Klasnja P. Micro-randomized trials: an experimental design for developing just-in-time adaptive interventions. Health Psychol. 2015;34:1220–8.
22. Vogelstein B, Kinzler KW. Cancer genes and the pathways they control. Nat Med. 2004;10 (8):789–99.
23. Kratchwill TR. Single subject research: strategies for evaluating change. Academic Press; 1978. p. 316.
24. Zucker DR, et al. Combining single patient (N-of-1) trials to estimate population treatment effects and to evaluate individual patient responses to treatment. J Clin Epidemiol. 1997;50 (4):401–10.
25. Joy TR, Zou GY, Mahon JL. N-of-1 (single-patient) trials for statin-related myalgia. Ann Intern Med. 2014;161(7):531–2.
26. Breivik H, et al. Assessment of pain. Br J Anaesth. 2008;101(1):17–24.
27. Marcolino MS, et al. The impact of mHealth interventions: systematic review of systematic reviews. JMIR Mhealth Uhealth. 2018;6(1):
28. Gurman TA, Rubin SE, Roess AA. Effectiveness of mHealth behavior change communication interventions in developing countries: a systematic review of the literature. J Health Commun. 2012;17(Suppl 1):82–104.
29. Devi BR, et al. mHealth: an updated systematic review with a focus on HIV/AIDS and tuberculosis long term management using mobile phones. Comput Methods Prog Biomed. 2015;122(2):257–65.
30. Sanders L. An evolving map of design practice and design research. Interactions. 2008;XV (6).
31. Kelders SM, et al. Evaluation of a web-based lifestyle coach designed to maintain a healthy bodyweight. J Telemed Telecare. 2010;16(1):3–7.
32. Wanner M, et al. Comparison of trial participants and open access users of a web-based physical activity intervention regarding adherence, attrition, and repeated participation. J Med Internet Res. 2010;12(1):
33. van Gemert-Pijnen JE, et al. A holistic framework to improve the uptake and impact of eHealth technologies. J Med Internet Res. 2011;13(4):
34. Tippey KG, Weinger MB. User-centered design means better patient care. Biomed Instrum Technol. 2017;51(3):220–2.
35. Jessen S, Mirkovic J, Ruland CM. Creating gameful design in mhealth: a participatory co-design approach. JMIR Mhealth Uhealth. 2018;6(12):
36. Zachary WW, et al. Participatory design of a social networking app to support type II diabetes self-management in low-income minority communities. Proc Int Symp Hum Factors Ergon Healthc. 2017;6(1):37–43.
37. Lamberti MJ, Getz K. White paper: Profiles of new approaches to improving the efficiency and performance of pharmaceutical drug development. Tufts Center for the Study of Drug Development, Boston, MA; 2015.
38. Sertkaya A, et al. Key cost drivers of pharmaceutical clinical trials in the United States. Clin Trials. 2016;13(2):117–26.

39. Ross S, et al. Barriers to participation in randomised controlled trials: a systematic review. J Clin Epidemiol. 1999;52(12):1143–56.
40. Covington D, Veley V. The remote patient-centered approach in clinical research. Appl Clin Trials. 2015.
41. Dorsey ER, et al. Novel methods and technologies for 21st-century clinical trials: a review. JAMA Neurol. 2015;72(5):582–8.
42. Europe's First Fully Remote Diabetes Trial.
43. ClinicalHealth Announces Successful Results for an Entirely Remote Online Clinical Trial. 2016.
44. Hirsch IB, et al. Incorporating site-less clinical trials into drug development: a framework for action. Clin Ther. 2017;39(5):1064–76.
45. Perez MV, et al. Large-scale assessment of a smartwatch to identify atrial fibrillation. N Engl J Med. 2019;381(20):1909–17.
46. Brown CA, Lilford RJ. The stepped wedge trial design: a systematic review. BMC Med Res Methodol. 2006;6:54.
47. Li YH, Mullette E, Brant JM. The stepped-wedge trial design: paving the way for cancer care delivery research. J Adv Pract Oncol. 2018;9(7):722–7.
48. Chapman AR, et al. High-sensitivity cardiac troponin and the universal definition of myocardial infarction. Circulation. 2020;141(3):161–71.

Shared Decision Making

David I. Feldman, Ramzi Dudum, and Roger S. Blumenthal

Shared Decision Making: The Introduction

Shared decision making is "an approach where clinicians and patients share the best available evidence when faced with the task of making decisions, and where patients are supported to consider options, to achieve informed preferences" [1]. Sir William Osler once said,

> "The good physician treats the disease; the great physician treats the patient who has the disease" [2].

When Osler practiced medicine, technology was rudimentary and accessing medical knowledge was difficult for even the savviest patients [3]. For these reasons, as well as an emphasis on paternalistic practice patterns [4], clinicians were the primary source of medical knowledge and were often trusted to make management decisions on behalf of patients. This agreement defined the clinician-patient relationship during that period.

The message of this quote continues to hold true, but the relationship between clinicians and patients has changed. Lifesaving, high quality care requires more than brilliant diagnosticians; it requires trust and effective communication, which are critical to building a healthy clinician-patient relationship. Once this occurs, and clinicians better understand the patient—who they are, their goals, their understanding, their unique personal situation that may impact the treatment alliance—then they can begin the process of shared decision making to treat the patient and their disease [5].

Shared decision making was first cited in 1982 to study the ethical problems in medicine and biochemical and behavioral research by the President's Commission [6]. Roughly a decade and a half later, Charles et al. recognized that the term had been poorly defined and largely underutilized; he proposed a model to help guide

D. I. Feldman (✉) · R. Dudum · R. S. Blumenthal
Baltimore, MD 21287, US
e-mail: dfeldm11@jhmi.edu

© Springer Nature Switzerland AG 2021

S. S. Martin (ed.), *Precision Medicine in Cardiovascular Disease Prevention*,
https://doi.org/10.1007/978-3-030-75055-8_8

individuals with life threatening or other serious illnesses who reached a crossroads in terms of treatment options [7].

The basis of this model required a clinician and a patient to share information that would help build a consensus about a preferred treatment option, which would then be implemented. Two years later, given the concern at the oversimplification of the shared decision-making process, Charles et al. addended the original framework to recognize the importance of flexibility throughout the process [8]. This would attempt to account for changes that may occur as the discussion or patient preferences evolved.

While shared decision making was first officially referenced as early as the 1980s, the principles, which focus on patient centered care, date back much further [6]. Like today, where both the Institute of Medicine [9] and the United States Preventive Services Task Force (USPSTF) [10] encourage clinicians to implement shared decision making in their practice to optimize health care decisions, Osler identified the utility of this early on in his practice [2].

Now more than ever though, with increased access to medical knowledge through the internet and social media, patients have clearly voiced their preference to be actively involved in the decision making process [11–13]. Incorporating this process into the daily practice of clinicians is not only important to protect patient autonomy but is critical to achieve optimal clinical outcomes [14].

The Role of Shared Decision Making in Personalizing Care

Cardiology, a field with decades of advancements helping to reduce the global burden of morbidity and mortality, abounds with decisions that require active participation of both clinicians and patients. Despite hundreds of methodologically rigorous randomized controlled clinical trials attempting to elucidate clinical uncertainties, many difficult or nuanced decisions such as the management of stable coronary artery disease, anticoagulation in atrial fibrillation, and placement of implantable cardioverter-defibrillators still exist. Each scenario requires clinicians to assess patient priorities, including the patient's prior experiences, perceived risk and potential benefits of therapy, and desire for autonomy.

Often patients are unable to accurately assess their personal risk of atherosclerotic cardiovascular disease (ASCVD) and when given the choice would prefer a "whatever the doctor or other clinician recommends" approach as long as they understand why the health care professional is making a certain recommendation [15]. Formulating the final recommendation requires the clinician to first have an accurate in-depth under-standing of the patient's cardiovascular risk profile and associated ASCVD risk, and then reconcile this with both clinical guidelines and clinical trial data. As with any informed consent process, while communicating the potential benefits of treatment is essential, a clinician must also explain the possible risks and alternatives to therapy. These key components of the clinician-patient discussion allow for more effective shared decision making in cardiovascular prevention.

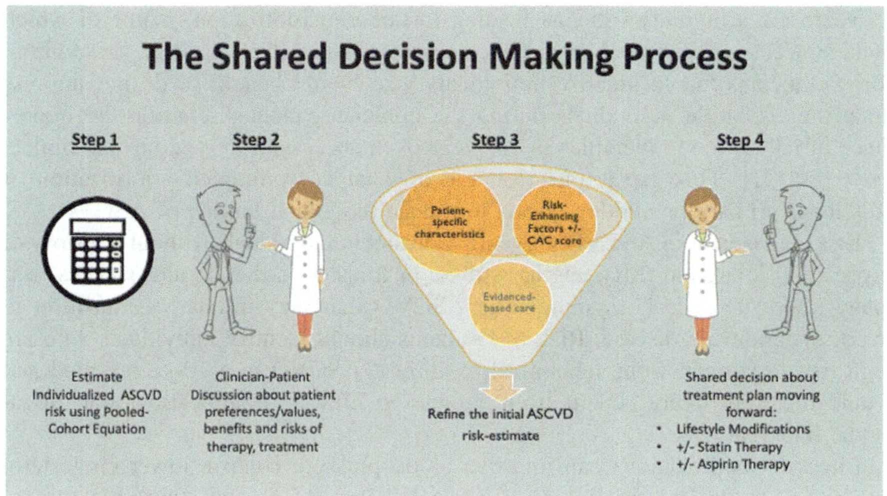

Fig. 1 The shared decision making process

Incorporating the shared decision making process into clinical practice has brought new meaning to personalized, precision medicine in the field of Cardiology (Fig. 1). In each clinical encounter, clinicians are tasked with disseminating accurate, understandable health information based on a patient's risk assessment and therapeutic options. During this discussion, a clinician will actively engage patients to explore their values and expectations of care to reach a shared path forward. It informs patients of the available treatment options and manages expectations, both of which improve individual understanding of the possible benefits and harms [16].

By stimulating patients' involvement in the decision making of their own care plan, clinicians are ensuring that the patient's personal values and choices are included. As a result of including patient preferences into the decision making process, clinicians help patient's think more positively about their disease process, better adhere to their treatment regimen, and feel more satisfied with their health outcomes [17, 18].

Shared Decision Making Highlighted in the ACC/AHA Guidelines

Despite major advancements in the understanding of the pathophysiology, diagnostic testing, and therapeutic armamentarium, cardiovascular disease remains the leading cause of death nationwide [19]. Even today, interventions like initiating statin therapy, which can slow or prevent disease progression in individuals without a history of ASCVD, are not being maximally utilized.

There are a myriad of factors leading to this underutilization—some of which include access and affordability of medicines and side effect profiles. In addition, some clinicians fail to identify individuals who would benefit or do not impress upon those eligible individuals during the clinician-patient discussion the importance of adherence to therapies that have proven successful in randomized clinical trials [20, 21]. This gap is one example of what has prompted prioritization of additional primary prevention efforts to reduce the global burden of ASCVD.

Risk assessment in ASCVD prevention occurs in individuals without a history of myocardial infarction (MI), angina, stroke, or transient ischemic attack. However, many have subclinical, asymptomatic ASCVD that may ultimately transition to overt, symptomatic disease. Risk assessments should identify individuals who are high risk to convert from subclinical to clinical ASCVD in a 10-year period and would therefore likely benefit from aggressive lifestyle modifications and therapeutic interventions.

Lifestyle modifications can improve blood pressure control, lower cholesterol levels, and reduce the risk for ASCVD or diabetes. As a result, these recommendations are unanimously first-line in all individuals at risk for ASCVD. Once diet and lifestyle habits are reviewed and recommendations regarding a heart healthy diet, regular aerobic exercise, maintenance of an ideal body weight, and avoidance of tobacco products are provided, then a clinician can discuss pharmacologic options and more intensified lifestyle changes for ASCVD risk reduction [22].

In 2013, the American College of Cardiology (ACC)/American Heart Association (AHA) Guideline on the Treatment of Blood Cholesterol to Reduce ASCVD Risk in Adults incorporated the principles of shared decision making into their model for whom to treat with statin therapy [23]. Shared decision making was integrated into the guidelines in order to best facilitate patient-centered care and customize appropriate preventive therapies to those most likely to benefit. Personalization becomes tantamount since each patient may have different baseline risk factors or lifestyle practices, could experience different side effects or adverse outcomes, and may feel differently about initiating statin therapy. Through optimizing therapeutic partnerships and alliances, shared decision making will more effectively reduce the global ASCVD burden.

Statin Use in Primary Prevention

Statin medications have been a mainstay when it comes to therapy for primary ASCVD prevention. Since the first statin was introduced to the market in 1987 (lovastatin) [24], it has been the primary goal of clinicians to responsibly allocate statins to individuals at high risk for ASCVD, where the benefits clearly outweigh the risks. Prior to the 2013 ACC/AHA cholesterol guidelines, treatment with statin therapy was determined based on low-density lipoprotein cholesterol (LDL-C) thresholds; an LDL-C that was above 'goal' required up-titration of the statin or addition of other non-statin lipid lowering therapies.

While LDL-C levels are important, the association with adverse cardiovascular events instead mirrors the estimated ASCVD risk [25]. In fact, roughly 35% of adverse events secondary to ASCVD occur in individuals with a total cholesterol < 200 mg/dl (this was the prior cut-off for normal total cholesterol levels), which suggests that ASCVD risk is multifactorial and adverse events can occur despite normal cholesterol levels [26]. However, the Cholesterol Treatment Trialists' Collaboration was transformative for demonstrating the wide-ranging benefits of statin therapy on LDL-C levels and ASCVD risk reduction; it highlighted that for every 39 mg/dl reduction in LDL-C the relative risk of incident ASCVD was also decreased by ~22% [27].

After publication of the 2013 cholesterol guidelines though, this concept of LDL-C goals was removed, and statin eligibility and intensity were primarily determined by the Pooled Cohort Equations (PCE) individualized risk assessment. If the guidelines were fully implemented, it was determined that the new statin prescribing pattern would broaden eligibility to >12 million newly identified high-risk primary prevention adults in the United States [28]. Given the heterogeneity among those individuals who would now qualify for statin therapy, determining individualized factors that can help inform the clinician-patient discussion and reclassify ASCVD risk was critical [29].

Therefore, each patient required their own individualized clinician-patient discussion about whether they would benefit from statin therapy to help reduce their risk for ASCVD. The importance of this discussion is emphasized frequently, knowing that the ultimate patient care decisions must be made together by the clinician and patient in light of the circumstances described by the patient [23]. This process, which describes shared decision making, is a critical part of the clinician-patient discussion.

The 2013 ACC/AHA cholesterol guidelines are an invaluable resource for referencing the highest quality clinical recommendations for reducing ASCVD risk. However, successful implementation of the guidelines in the primary prevention setting requires more than optimal interpretation and seamless application of the recommendations into clinical practice [30]. With the evolution and prioritization of patient autonomy and a shift from paternalism, successful implementation requires special attention to the clinician-patient risk discussion.

During this discussion, clinicians should individualize risk assessment and the potential for risk reduction, clarify the possibility for adverse effects or drug-drug interactions, and incorporate patient preferences. Only then can clinicians strengthen their relationship with patients. Once a patient's personal preferences are incorporated and the patient is maximally engaged to increase adherence, then clinicians and patients together can decide on a strategy that will optimize an individual's 10-year and 30-year risk for ASCVD.

Shared Decision Making: The Transition from the Population to Individual Level

In pursuit of optimal primary prevention of ASCVD, clinicians and policymakers are tasked with navigating the most effective strategy—should focus be placed on population-level, public health, and structural interventions or targeting individuals at highest risk for disease? Geoffrey Rose, a British epidemiologist, observed the interplay between risk at the individual and population level noting that, "a large number of people at a small risk may give rise to more cases of disease than the small number who are a high risk" [31].

Rose went on to describe that individual level risk variance may be "inherent in genes, behavior, and social factors" [31], whereas population level disease incidence may not be predicted by these same factors [32]. As such, Rose described the importance of intervening with a "population strategy" in addition to the traditional "high-risk strategy" [32].

In cardiovascular prevention, a population strategy has yielded significant improvement in ASCVD risk by reducing exposure to certain well-known risk factors—including tobacco products, sugar sweetened beverages, processed foods, and environmental pollutants [33]. It also has been instrumental in increasing access to health promoting behaviors—including increased physical activity by developing more walkable, safe cities, decreasing sedentary behavior by introducing active workstations in the professional environment, and incentivizing the distribution of fresh foods to food deserts [33]. Together, these interventions have had major effects on our population's ASCVD risk and for many individuals may have proven sufficient to reduce downstream ASCVD events [34].

While professional organizations and policymakers are drivers for implementing change at the population level, individual clinicians are uniquely suited to implement change at the individual level. At this level, clinicians can target both those at low and intermediate risk, as well as those at higher risk using the PCE [35]. In 2013, Goff et al. provided clinicians with this updated individualized risk assessment tool that would serve as the backbone for bringing epidemiologic observations to the individual [35].

Through the utilization of cohort-level prediction tools, appropriate ASCVD risk reduction begins with accurate risk assessment, which facilitates patient centered care by way of a clinician-patient risk discussion, and ultimately a shared decision on a treatment strategy. In 2013, the demand for this individualized approach to ASCVD risk reduction was identified by guideline writers who explicitly incorporated clinician-patient discussions and shared decision making into their recommendations.

Shared Decision Making in Clinical Practice

In practice, a clinician should calculate the 10-year ASCVD risk with the PCE for individuals 40 to 75 years of age, without clinical ASCVD or diabetes with a LDL-C level of 70 to 189 mg/dl [23]. Individual risk estimation is then completed every 4 to 6 years and should not be used again in patients already started on statins or in individuals immediately following a short course of lifestyle modifications [23].

Initiating statin therapy is a Class of Recommendation (COR) I, Level of Evidence (LOE) A recommendation when a patient has clinical ASCVD, diabetes and an LDL-C between 70–189 mg/dl, or an estimated 10-year ASCVD risk of 7.5% and an LDL-C between 70–189 mg/dl. There is also a COR I, LOE B recommendation when a patient has primary LDL-C $\geq$ 190 mg/dl (Fig. 2) [23]. The threshold to recommend starting statin therapy in these groups was based on a number need to treat to prevent an ASCVD event versus the number needed to potentially harm (with respect to diabetes or other side effects) analysis. However, given that statins are commonly a lifelong medication, the guideline authors emphasized the central role for a clinician-patient discussion, which can facilitate shared decision making.

To ensure all aspects of the clinician-patient discussion were addressed before deciding to prescribe a statin, a checklist was developed and required all criteria to be met before appropriateness of statin therapy is determined [30]. Table 1 is an adapted version of the checklist, which includes pertinent updates since the publication of the original manuscript. Incorporating the checklist into clinical practice provides another layer of protection to ensure that the guideline recommendations take into account patient specific factors and preferences.

A Guideline Driven Approach to Statin Therapy

Statin Therapy Benefit Groups	Class of Recommendation	Level of Evidence
Clinical Atherosclerotic Cardiovascular Disease	Class I	Level of Evidence A
Primary Low-Density Lipoprotein Cholesterol $\geq$190 mg/dL	Class I	Level of Evidence B
Diabetes and a Low-Density Lipoprotein Cholesterol between 70 – 189 mg/dL	Class I	Level of Evidence A
10-year Atherosclerotic Cardiovascular Disease Risk $\geq$7.5% and a Low-Density Lipoprotein Cholesterol between 70 – 189 mg/dL	Class I	Level of Evidence A

Fig. 2 A guideline driven approach to statin therapy

Table 1 Checklist for the clinician-patient risk discussion

Checklist for clinician-patient risk discussion
Calculate the individual 10-year or 30-year ASCVD risk using the ACC/AHA Pooled Cohort Equations
Discuss all of the lifestyle and pharmacologic options for risk reduction using the 'ABCDE' approach to ASCVD prevention:
– *Aspirin*
– *Blood pressure*
– *Cholesterol*
– *Cigarette smoking*
– *Diet*
– *Diabetes control*
– *Exercise*
Consider an individual's ASCVD REF for personalized risk assessment
Refine risk using objective assessments of an individual's risk for ASCVD (i.e., CAC score)
Optimize aggressive behavioral and lifestyle modifications
Assess willingness to start medications to maximize risk reduction
Discuss the benefits and potential side effects of statin therapy (first line) for ASCVD risk reduction
Encourage patient involvement in the decision making process by incorporating individualized values and preferences
Answer specific questions regarding the individualized approach to ASCVD risk reduction
Reassess at each subsequent clinician patient encounter

Abbreviations: ASCVD, atherosclerotic cardiovascular disease; ACC, American College of Cardiology; AHA, American Heart Association; REF, Risk Enhancing Factor; CAC, Coronary Artery Calcium

While individual risk can help stratify patients into specific subgroups for determining appropriate treatment options, it should serve as a starting point to begin the discussion and decision making process [36]. When this process is not prioritized or ignored completely [37, 38], patients may become disengaged, the treatment alliance can break down, and outcomes may be worse [14].

Shared Decision Making—Discussing Patient Risk

To help increase the likelihood that shared decision making occurs among clinicians and patients, the 2013 ACC/AHA cholesterol guideline committee developed the ACC/AHA Risk Estimator Application. It is widely available, easily accessible, and now even incorporated into many electronic medical records. This facilitated patients seeing firsthand the data that went into calculating a 10-year ASCVD risk score. It also allowed them to see how adjustments in their risk factor profiles impacted the estimation of their 10-year ASCVD risk.

For example, in an otherwise healthy 50-year-old African American male, transitioning from a smoker to non-smoker decreases his 10-year ASCVD risk on the application from 9 to 5%, respectively. Depending on an individual's 10-year ASCVD risk or 30-year risk (calculated in those 20 to 59 years of age through an alternative algorithm [39]), it personalizes therapeutic and lifestyle guideline recommendations relevant to the individual risk factor profile and 10-year or lifetime risk for ASCVD. In the gentleman whose case is described above, utilizing just the lifestyle modifications, including a recommendation to stop smoking, can alter his estimated ASCVD risk from intermediate to borderline risk.

This resource was pivotal in helping to communicate the concept of risk to patients, a topic often perceived as difficult to understand by both patients and clinicians, alike. Many variables can affect how risk is perceived, including how clinicians communicate risk, the trust a patient has in his/her clinician, and the nature of the risk communicated (i.e. imminent versus abstract) [40]. A number of these variables can decrease the perceived ASCVD risk—including that heart disease is often viewed as a chronic rather than catastrophic condition, the familiarity with which people view heart disease and its associated complications, and the perception of control over the disease and the risk factors, to name a few [40].

In its simplest form, risk is often perceived as the "the probability of something bad happening" [41]. The ways in which this is presented can greatly impact how patients view their individual risk. For instance, one example (others are listed in Table 2) to communicate risk using our patient described above with an initial 10-year ASCVD risk of $\sim$ 9% would be to have a physician say, "of 100 patients like you, 9 would be expected to have a stroke or heart attack in the next 10 years [30, 42]. The corollary to this, would be to state that there is a roughly 90% chance that the patient does not have a stroke or heart attack over the next 10 years. A positive versus a negative framing can greatly change how risk is perceived [43].

For our 50 year-old gentleman who is a current smoker, the way we frame his choice to become a non-smoker, could also shift how he views the magnitude of effect. Rather than saying that smoking cessation could decrease his risk of stroke or heart disease by 4% over the next 10 years, a better way to frame this, which might be more likely to change his behavior, would be to say that he could reduce his risk of stroke or heart disease over the next 10-years by over 40% with smoking cessation [44]. Other ways to communicate risk employ the incorporation of visual cues, which could show absolute risk and incremental benefits/risks associated with drug therapy using risk pictographs [45].

With multiple options available for conveying risk to patients, a systematic review was completed to try and elucidate whether one method was superior. While the review did not identify the optimal method for conveying risk, it suggested that incorporating visual cues leads to improved patient understanding and satisfaction [46]. The significance of clearly conveying risk to patients during the clinician-patient discussion is that when embarking on the process of shared

Table 2 Options for conveying risk during a clinician-patient discussion

Options for conveying risk during a clinician-patient discussion	
Recommendation:	*Rationale:*
Start by having a patient estimate their own risk	Patients may have optimistic or pessimistic biases which may require different communication strategies
Communicate risk using visual cues	Visual cues lead to improved patient understanding and satisfaction
Optimize the use of both absolute risk reduction and relative risk reduction	Patients may have difficulty justifying a daily medication for a 2% absolute risk reduction however they may be more inclined to adhere if it is framed as a 40% relative risk reduction
Determine whether qualitative or quantitative expression of risk is preferred	When informing a patient they are high risk, some patients will respond more to hearing "high risk" for adverse events in a 10-year period compared to others who may prefer >20% risk for adverse events in a 10-year period
Utilize both 10 and 30-year risk estimates when applicable	In high risk young adults, lifetime risk for an adverse event may be more impactful. For example, in the next 10 years, your risk for a myocardial infarction is 10% vs. you have a >50% chance of having a myocardial infarction in your lifetime
When conveying risk, provide both the positive and negative perspective	A positive (there is a >90% chance you do not have a myocardial infarction) versus a negative (of 100 people like you, 9 would be expected to have a myocardial infarction) framing can greatly change how risk is perceived

decision making, patients have been given the information necessary to make informed decisions about their treatment plan.

When Shared Decision Making Feels Like Shared Decision Guessing

While the 2013 cholesterol guidelines successfully identified the majority of individuals who would benefit from statin therapy after engaging in a clinician-patient discussion, there are certain groups where treatment decisions regardless of the most effective clinician-patient discussions are uncertain. After estimating an individual's ASCVD risk using the PCE, four discrete groups clearly benefit from statin initiation after a clinician-patient discussion: (1) individuals with clinical ASCVD, (2) individuals with LDL-C $\geq$ 190 mg/dl, (3) individuals aged 40–75 years old + diabetes + LDL-C 70–189 mg/dl, and (4) individuals with 10-year ASCVD risk $\geq$ 7.5% + LDL-C 70–189 mg/dl.

The first three subgroups are based on objective data and therefore agreeing on a treatment plan after a clear explanation of the risk and perceived benefit of treatment often occurs. The fourth group—10-year ASCVD risk $\geq$ 7.5% + LDL-C 70–189 mg/dl—relies on the accuracy of the PCE, which performs poorly in certain subgroups of the population. For instance, in individuals with low socioeconomic status, human immunodeficiency virus, or inflammatory diseases including systemic lupus erythematosus or rheumatoid arthritis, the PCE often underestimates the 10-year ASCVD risk [47]. In highly engaged, high socioeconomic status individuals, the PCE overestimates the 10-year ASCVD risk [48].

The relevance of this issue dates back to when the 2013 cholesterol guideline was published, and many clinicians felt certain individuals fell into subgroups where the recommendations were less clear based on uncertainty about the accuracy of the risk estimation. In fact, in many United States cohorts, observed ASCVD event rates were much lower than expected rates, which leads to overtreatment with statin therapy and possibly aspirin or antihypertensive therapy [49].

In 2019, when the ACC/AHA Guideline on the Primary Prevention of ASCVD was published, the approach to identifying individuals who would benefit from statin initiation was modified [50]. Previously, individuals with a 10-year ASCVD risk of <5% (low risk) and $\geq$ 20% (high risk) were prescribed aggressive lifestyle modifications only and aggressive lifestyle modification and drug therapy after a clinician-patient discussion, respectively. However, now borderline (5–7.5%) and intermediate (7.5–20%) risk individuals should engage in a clinician-patient discussion that considers risk enhancing factors and the net benefit of therapy.

When the decision to start statin therapy is uncertain, risk enhancing factors can help provide clearer evidence of individual ASCVD risk and can guide decisions around preventive therapy. While the list of risk enhancing factors is expansive, including family history of premature ASCVD, the presence of metabolic syndrome, chronic kidney disease, chronic inflammatory conditions, premature menopause, or high-risk race/ethnicities, they were compiled to help further risk stratify the need for preventive interventions (e.g., statin therapy) when initial risk-based decisions were uncertain. For example, when the PCE provide an ASCVD risk that lands in the broad intermediate risk range and the treatment decisions are uncertain, start by determining the presence of risk enhancing factors. When present, these risk enhancing factors can shift initial risk estimates to ensure more appropriate treatment intensity [51].

Selective Use of Coronary Artery Calcium Measurements

As part of this shared decision making process, clinicians can also offer a coronary artery calcium (CAC) scan, which helps reclassify individual risk either upward or downward. A CAC score can reclassify risk in both the borderline and intermediate risk groups but generally does not meaningfully alter risk in both the low and high-risk groups [52]; one exception may involve those with a family history of premature ASCVD [53]. Certain risk enhancing factors were emphasized including the use of CAC scores, which as a single risk enhancing factor to guide clinician-patient risk discussion received a COR IIa, LOE B-NR.

Singling out CAC scores from the large list of risk enhancing factors is based on decades of research that demonstrate its strong graded association with 10-year risk of ASCVD [54]. Increased CAC scores are associated with a tenfold higher risk of ASCVD events on top of traditional cardiovascular risk factors as compared to a person with no CAC and comparable risk factors [55]. However, when CAC is absent, there is a very low 10–15-year risk for future ASCVD events and patients can opt for lifestyle modifications with shared decision making that focuses on flexible treatment goals [56].

Importantly, CAC also accurately predicts ASCVD risk independent of age, race, and sex, which allows for broad application of risk prediction [54]. Once a CAC score is determined in the borderline and intermediate risk individuals who are undecided on therapy or there is clinical uncertainty regarding the net benefit of statin therapy, the risk revision process can begin. If negative (CAC = 0), CAC scores can help reassure individuals that their risk for an adverse event in the next 5 years is low despite statin therapy [57]. Therefore, the patient is below the threshold for statin benefit, and after a clinician-patient discussion, avoidance or postponement of drug therapy is reasonable.

If CAC is 1–99 and <75th percentile for age, sex and race, the clinician-patient discussion can now include objective evidence that subclinical atherosclerosis is present, and while the risk estimate is roughly similar to what was estimated by the PCE initially, a more informed decision can be made whether to initiate statin therapy or postpone with plans to repeat CAC testing in ~ 5 years. In these cases, CAC can also be used as a motivational tool that objectively demonstrates subclinical atherosclerosis and further informs the individual regarding his/her ASCVD risk and benefit of therapy.

If CAC is >100, the patient is clearly above the threshold for statin benefit, and after a clinician-patient discussion and shared decision making, statin therapy should be initiated. While CAC is not meant to be a screening test to determine an individual's eligibility for statin therapy, it can be helpful in selective cases in determining how aggressive a clinician should be in initiating treatment in a patient. Once treatment is initiated, CAC can also affect behavioral motivation and medication adherence [58]. In fact, individuals with elevated CAC scores typically are more likely to initiate and adhere to lifestyle and pharmacologic interventions for ASCVD risk reduction [59, 60].

When 'Plan A' Fails, Lean on Shared Decision Making

"It is much more important to know what sort of a patient has a disease than what sort of a disease a patient has."

—Sir William Osler

Identifying individuals at risk for ASCVD is easier with tools like the PCE. After shared decision making, many individuals can lower their ASCVD risk through aggressive lifestyle modifications and initiation of statin therapy. However, roughly 10–15% of people are intolerant to their first statin therapy and an even greater percentage are hesitant to start statin therapy, which typically is a lifetime medication [61].

Statin Associated Side-Effects

When the shared decision making process leads to the initiation of statin therapy, those individuals who do not tolerate the medication and report adverse side effects of the drug will generally be unable to adhere to therapy [62]. It is critical that despite the initial side effects of statin therapy, that the clinician and patient attempt alternatives to the initial statin prescription such as taking a statin that may be hydrophilic (e.g. rosuvastatin), taking a lower intensity statin, or taking the statin every other day or even weekly.

A patient cannot be considered completely statin intolerant until patients have tried multiple statins, weekly dosing and have clear documentation of new symptoms from baseline since starting the medication. There are alternative treatments to help lower LDL-C and overall ASCVD risk in patients who are ultimately deemed statin intolerant.

Ezetimibe, PCSK9-Inhibitors, Icosapent Ethyl & Bempedoic Acid

Ezetimibe reduces intestinal absorption of cholesterol and reduces LDL-C and ASCVD outcomes when added on top of statin therapy [63]. For this reason, in addition to its excellent safety profile over 7 years of follow-up, it is often added to maximally tolerated statin therapy for those highest risk individuals and in those high-risk individuals who cannot tolerate low dose or weekly dosing of statin therapy. The latter group represents a subpopulation of at-risk individuals who could benefit from the ASCVD risk reduction of statin therapy, but report statin associated muscle symptoms such as myalgia, myopathy or rarely rhabdomyolysis. Since publication of the Improved Reduction of Outcomes: Vytorin Efficacy

International Trial (IMPROVE-IT), ezetimibe has been increasingly prescribed in statin intolerant patients who could benefit from further LDL-C lowering therapy.

When statin intolerant patients have a high baseline ASCVD risk (ASCVD risk >20%, CAC score >100), the risk reduction benefits of ezetimibe alone are often not sufficient. Proprotein convertase subtilisin/kexin type 9 inhibitors (PCSK9-I) were first FDA approved in 2015 as an option for additional LDL-C reduction on top of high-intensity statin [64]. Since then, in addition to the LDL-C lowering effects, it has proven to reduce ASCVD outcomes when added to a moderate/high intensity statin.

In current practice, PCSK9-I are being utilized in high-risk individuals on maximally tolerated statin and LDL-C $\geq$ 70 mg/dl. However, the implications of this drug and its drastic ASCVD risk reduction capabilities are revolutionary for those individuals at high ASCVD risk who are unable to tolerate statin therapy secondary to reported side effects. When comparing the side effect profile for PCSK9-I and placebo, the rate of both minor and serious adverse events was similar, and therefore PCSK9-I are not only effective at reducing risk but generally very well tolerated.

In 2019, icosapent ethyl, which is a highly purified eicosapentaenoic acid ethyl ester, was studied in individuals with established cardiovascular disease or with diabetes and other risk factors who had already been initiated on statin therapy [65]. Individuals had to have a triglyceride level of 135 to 499 mg/dl and an LDL-C level of 40 to 100 mg/dl. Those individuals who were randomized to icosapent ethyl had lower triglycerides and fewer cardiovascular events and cardiovascular deaths. They also experienced a small increase in hospitalizations for atrial fibrillation or flutter and serious bleeding events. While icosapent ethyl is a non-LDL-C lowering therapy, it has a significant role in reducing adverse cardiovascular events and therefore should be considered in all individuals at risk for ASCVD, including in those who are unable to tolerate statin therapy.

Bempedoic acid—a nonstatin LDL-C lowering therapy that targets the cholesterol biosynthesis pathway upstream of statin therapy via inhibition of adenosine triphosphate-citrate lyase—is orally administered as a prodrug and later converted to its active form by a hepatic enzyme not present in skeletal muscles. As a promising therapy for patients with statin-associated muscle symptoms, its efficacy and safety were first demonstrated in statin-intolerant patients who required additional LDL-C lowering in both the Cholesterol Lowering via Bempedoic Acid, an ACL-Inhibiting Regimen (CLEAR) Tranquility and Serenity trials [66, 67].

In the CLEAR Wisdom and Harmony trials, its efficacy and safety were assessed in high-risk cardiovascular patients with ASCVD, heterozygous familial hypercholesterolemia (HeFH) or both. In individuals on maximally tolerated statin therapy, addition of bempedoic acid resulted in $\sim$ 18% LDL-C lowering compared to placebo [68, 69]. When studied in combination with ezetimibe in a similar high-risk population on maximally tolerated statin, LDL-C lowering reached upwards of 40% compared to placebo [70].

The side-effect profile of bempedoic acid did not differ substantially from the placebo subgroup, however the incidence of adverse events leading to discontinuation of the regimen was higher in bempedoic acid group, as was the incidence of gout [69]. Despite ongoing evaluation for its role on ASCVD events in the CLEAR Outcomes trial, the FDA approved its use in 2020 as an adjunct to diet and maximally tolerated statin therapy in adults with HeFH or established ASCVD who require additional LDL-C lowering [71, 72]. The FDA also approved a fixed-dose combination of bempedoic acid (180 mg) and ezetimibe (10 mg) for the same indications.

While statins are still first line for ASCVD risk reduction, ezetimibe, PCSK9-I, icosapent ethyl and bempedoic acid are helpful additions in high risk individuals or alternatives in statin intolerant patients. Most importantly, they are very well tolerated with limited side effect profiles.

Shared Decision Making Beyond Statins and LDL-C Lowering Therapies

Aspirin

In addition to statin therapy, aspirin was another cornerstone for the primary prevention of ASCVD for many years. After the AHA and USPSTF referenced its utility in their 2002 guidelines, it became one of the most commonly used medications for the primary prevention of ASCVD. In fact, in 2016, it was estimated that 40% of adults over 50 years of age in the United States were taking aspirin for the primary prevention of ASCVD [73]. These recommendations were based on data from studies like the Physicians' Heart Study (PHS), Thrombosis Prevention Trial (TPT), and Hypertension Optimal Trial (HOT) [74–76].

Using these data, the USPSTF conducted a meta-analysis to determine the effect of aspirin therapy on cardiovascular outcomes. In individuals with 5-year CVD risk between 3–5% (which equates to ~6–10% ASCVD risk), aspirin therapy resulted in 4–20 fewer coronary heart disease (CHD) events per 1000 person-years, at the cost of only 2–4 major gastrointestinal bleeding events per 1000-person years [77]. Later, in 2009, using data from the Women's Health Study, the USPSTF broadened the aspirin benefit group to include all men aged 45 to 79 and women aged 55 to 79 in order to reduce MI and strokes respectively, assuming the CVD risk was greater than the bleeding risk [78].

Since these initial recommendations, as the implementation of primary prevention efforts has improved in cardiology, the utility of aspirin in primary prevention has been questioned. In 2014, a meta-analysis was completed that demonstrated a modest but statistically significant reduction in events with aspirin for the primary prevention of ASCVD. However, the same study also identified a significantly increased risk of major bleeding. It was determined that over a 7-year period, 284 individuals needed to be treated with aspirin to prevent 1 major ASCVD event and 299 individuals needed to be treated to cause 1 major bleed [79].

After these data were published, a practical stepwise approach to the use of aspirin in primary prevention was proposed [80]. In those individuals with a 10-year ASCVD risk <10%, the bleeding risk outweighed the ASCVD risk reduction benefit. If the 10-year ASCVD risk was 10% or greater, the benefit of aspirin therapy depends on careful consideration of the individual's bleeding risk. If the patient had a history of bleeding without reversible causes or concurrent use of other medication that increase bleeding risk, the ASCVD risk reduction benefit from aspirin was thought to be insufficient to risk a major bleeding event. If there were no significant bleeding risk factors and the ASCVD risk was 10% or greater, individuals were recommended to initiate aspirin with caution (Fig. 3) [80].

In 2018, three trials studying aspirin in primary ASCVD prevention were published: the ASCEND (A Study of Cardiovascular Events in Diabetes) trial, the ARRIVE (Aspirin to Reduce Risk of Initial Vascular Events) trial, and the ASPREE (Aspirin in Reducing Events in the Elderly) trial [81–83]. In the ASCEND trial, which was enriched with primary prevention patients with diabetes, the number needed to treat to avoid a serious vascular event was lower than the number needed to harm to cause a major a bleed [81]. However, the overall benefit of prophylactic aspirin in primary prevention was less than demonstrated in trials over a decade ago where individuals were not optimized on other ASCVD preventive treatments, including hypertension and cholesterol therapies.

Given the mixed signal for ASCVD risk reduction with aspirin initiation and a significant harm signal in some individuals, all clinicians should engage their patients in shared decision making to ensure the patients values and preferences are considered before starting long-term aspirin therapy. The 2019 ACC/AHA Guideline on the Primary Prevention of Cardiovascular Disease emphasizes the need for an individualized assessment for the benefit of aspirin therapy in primary

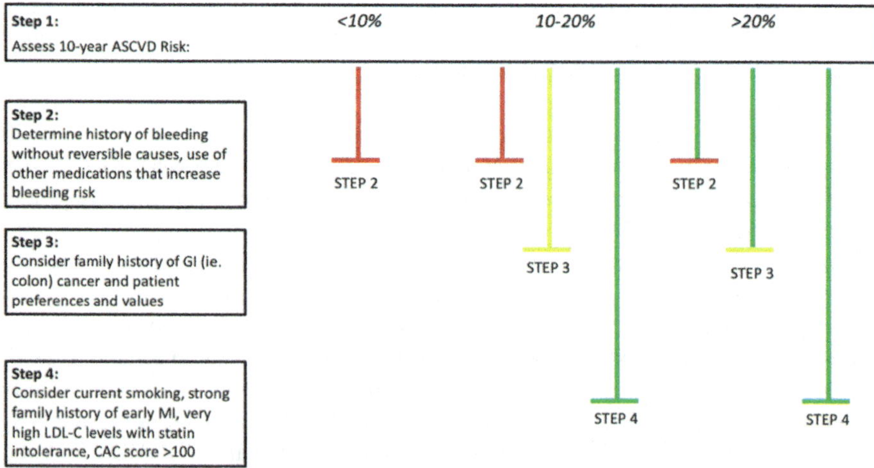

Fig. 3 Decision tree for aspirin therapy in ASCVD prevention

prevention [84]. They indicate the possible harm in those adults greater than 70 years of age who are at increased risk of bleeding.

In primary prevention, there is a COR IIB, LOE A recommendation for low-dose aspirin in select adults 40–70 years of age who are at higher ASCVD risk but not at increased bleeding risk [83]. Ultimately, thoughtful decisions are needed in the context of a clinician-patient risk discussion where factors such as current smoking, strong family history of early MI, very high LDL-C levels with statin intolerance, CAC score >100, and ASCVD risk >20% can be considered to determine the suitability of aspirin in primary ASCVD prevention [85].

Blood Pressure

Another key component to address ASCVD risk based on the PCE is blood pressure control. Based on an individual's systolic and diastolic blood pressure and current anti-hypertensive medication regimen, the Risk Estimator Application will provide standardized recommendations for blood pressure control as part of the ASCVD risk reduction process. As part of a clinician-patient risk discussion, individuals should consider initiating lifestyle and pharmacologic interventions including thiazide diuretics, angiotensin converting enzyme inhibitors (ACE-I), angiotensin II receptor blockers (ARB) or calcium channel blockers to help obtain better blood pressure control.

In adults with elevated blood pressure that may require anti-hypertensive medications, it is important to first ensure non-pharmacologic interventions are discussed during the shared decision making process. These non-pharmacologic options include weight loss, a heart-healthy diet, sodium reduction, dietary potassium supplementation, increased physical activity, and limiting alcohol [86].

The 2017 AHA/ACC Blood Pressure Guideline includes ranges of normal, elevated, high stage 1, and high stage 2 blood pressure, which is accompanied by recommendations for appropriate therapy based on the perceived risk [86]. While the Systolic Blood Pressure Intervention Trial (SPRINT) demonstrated a significant benefit ($\sim$25% relative risk reduction) of strict blood pressure control (target less than 120/80 versus less than 140/90) on the risk of MI, strokes, heart failure, or death, many clinicians will still target a more modest blood pressure (less than 130/80) given the potential for adverse events with more aggressive control [87].

Shared decision making is required to incorporate an individual's ASCVD risk and appropriately measured blood pressure to determine the most optimal combination of both lifestyle and pharmacologic interventions. In fact, these recommendations will differ depending on an individual's age, race, and cardiovascular risk factor profile.

For example, an African American patient with a 10-year ASCVD risk score 10% and a blood pressure $\geq$ 130/80 would benefit from a medication like a thiazide diuretic or calcium channel blocker for blood pressure control. If the same patient were Caucasian, the recommendation for optimal treatment would include thiazide diuretics (chlorthalidone preferred), calcium channel blockers, ACE-I or ARB. In all patients treated with anti-hypertensive medication, reliable screening for adverse signs or symptoms related to their treatment should be completed, and can include hypotension, syncope, bradycardia, electrolyte abnormalities, falls, or kidney damage [86].

Anticoagulation

While the ACC/AHA risk estimator application only references statin, aspirin and blood pressure medications as therapeutic options for ASCVD risk reduction in individuals, many other risk factors contribute to an individual's risk for ASCVD. Atrial fibrillation, which is the most common cardiac arrhythmia, is one important ASCVD risk factor not included in the PCE. Given the increasing prevalence and known harmful effects of atrial fibrillation including stroke and death, optimal risk reduction is important for preventing adverse outcomes. The cornerstone of treatment in atrial fibrillation is anticoagulation with vitamin K antagonist like warfarin or non-vitamin K antagonist oral anticoagulants (NOAC) like dabigatran, apixaban, rivaroxaban or edoxaban [88].

Shared decision making in the treatment of atrial fibrillation starts with calculating an individual's CHA_2DS_2-VASc score. This tool, which estimates the risk of ischemic stroke by considering the individual's age, sex, and history of congestive heart failure, hypertension, diabetes, stroke/TIA/thromboembolism, and vascular disease (MI, peripheral arterial disease, or aortic atherosclerosis), has demonstrated a graded association with score and risk for ischemic stroke.

For example, individuals with a CHA_2DS_2-VASc score of 0 have a $\sim 0.2\%$ risk for stroke each year; CHA_2DS_2-VASc score of 2 have a 2.2% risk for stroke each year; and CHA_2DS_2-VASc score of 9 have a 12.2% risk for stroke each year. Therefore, guidelines currently recommend individuals with atrial fibrillation and with a history of stroke or CHA_2DS_2-VASc of 2 or greater start on warfarin or a NOAC (assuming they have non-valvular atrial fibrillation) to reduce the risk for stroke [88].

Shared decision making in the setting of a clinician-patient discussion must occur prior to initiating anticoagulation because there is a known risk of bleeding from these medications. Similar to how the CHA_2DS_2-VASc score informs the benefit of anticoagulation for atrial fibrillation, the HAS-BLED score estimates risk of major bleeding in individuals on anticoagulation for atrial fibrillation [89].

Using this tool, the risk of bleeding is estimated using a validation study [90], and depending on the risk, a recommendation for anticoagulation is given. Based on the individual risk factors, including hypertension, renal or liver disease, stroke history, prior bleeding event, age, INR lability, alcohol use, and the use of other blood thinning medications, a score is given with an accompanying recommendation. If the score is less than or equal to 1/9 anticoagulation should be considered; 2/9 anticoagulation can be considered; and >3/9 alternatives to anticoagulation should be recommended as the individual has a very high bleeding risk [89, 90]. Controlling a patient's modifiable risk factors for atrial fibrillation (e.g. weight/body mass index/ waist circumference, alcohol intake, blood pressure, and obstructive sleep apnea) can help reduce the incidence of the disease and associated risk of treatment.

Like other decisions in cardiology, the management of anticoagulation in patients with atrial fibrillation requires an individualized clinician patient discussion focused on shared decision making. While some individuals may identify a daily or twice daily medication as an insignificant price to pay for stroke prevention, others may be interested in undergoing a one-time procedure like a left atrial appendage closure to eliminate the risk of stroke associated with atrial fibrillation. Ultimately, clinicians and patients must form an alliance, which allows for decisions to be made based on the the highest quality of evidence assuming it fits within the patient goals and preferences, in order to achieve maximal ASCVD risk reduction.

Conclusion

As medicine has evolved, so too has the clinician-patient relationship. What was once a more paternalistic and uniform practice pattern, has fortunately shifted to a more individualized and patient-oriented approach. In this new framework, the heart of primary prevention is centered around risk estimation using the PCE followed by a thoughtful clinician-patient discussion with the expressed purpose of engaging in shared decision making. In fact, many tools have been created to help guide and elucidate the best ways to communicate risk and the effects of behavioral modification. Effectively conveying risk to patients during the clinician-patient discussion substantiates the shared decision making process by providing patients the necessary information to make informed decisions about their treatment plan.

Utilizing a shared decision making approach allows the clinician to provide evidence-based recommendations for risk reduction and treatment that reflect the patient's values, goals, and concerns. When necessary, clinicians can opt for additional decision making aids such as risk-enhancing factors like coronary artery calcium, which can further inform the shared decision making process. Ultimately, this approach will better engage and empower patients in their cardiovascular care, which will likely lead to improved adherence to therapies and reduction in ASCVD risk and adverse events.

References

1. Elwyn G, Frosch D, Thomson R, et al. Shared decision making: a model for clinical practice. J Gen Intern Med. 2012;27(10):1361–7.
2. Centor RM. To be a great physician, you must understand the whole story. MedGenMed. 2007;9(1):59.

3. Hess EP, Coylewright M, Frosch DL, Shah ND. Implementation of shared decision making in cardiovascular care: past, present, and future. Circ Cardiovasc Qual Outcomes. 2014;7:797–803.

4. Siegler M. The progression of medicine: from physician paternalism to patient autonomy to bureaucratic parsimony. Arch Intern Med. 1985;145(4):713–5.

5. Hoffmann TC, Légaré F, Simmons MB, et al. Shared decision making: what do clinicians need to know and why should they bother? Med J Aust. 2014;201:35–9.

6. President' Commision for the Study of Ethical Problems in Medicine and Biomedical and Behavioral Research. Making health care decision: the ethical and legal implications of informed consent in the patient-practitioner relationship. US Code Annot US. 1982, 42: 300v.

7. Charles C, Gafni A, Whelan T. Shared decision-making in the medical encounter: what does it mean? (or it takes at least two to tango). Soc Sci Med. 1997;44:681–92.

8. Charles C, Gafni A, Whelan T. Decision-making in the physician-patient encounter: revisiting the shared treatment decision-making model. Soc Sci Med. 1999; 49:651–61.

9. Berwick DM. A user's manual for the IOM's 'Quality Chasm' report. Health Aff (Millwood). 2002;21(3):80–90.

10. Sheridan S, Harris R, Woolf S. Shared decision making about screening and chemoprevention. a suggested approach from the U.S Preventive Services Task Force. American Journal of Preventive Medicine. 2004;26(1):56–66

11. Deber RB, Kraetschmer N, Irvine J. What role do patients wish to play in treatment decision making? Arch Int Med. 1996;156:1414–20.

12. Adams JR, Elwyn G, Légaré F, Frosch DL. Communicating with physicians about medical decisions: a reluctance to disagree. Arch Intern Med. 2012;172:1184–6.

13. Krumholz HM, Barreto-Filho JA, Jones PG, Li Y, Spertus JA. Decision-making preferences among patients with an acute myocardial infarction. JAMA Intern Med. 2013;173:1252–7.

14. Kaplan SH, Greenfield S, Ware JE. Assessing the effects of physician-patient interactions on the outcomes of chronic disease. Med Care. 1989;27(3 suppl):S110–2.

15. van der Weijden T, van Steenkiste B, Stoffers HE, et al. Primary prevention of cardiovascular diseases in general practice: mismatch between cardiovascular risk and patients' risk perceptions. Med Dec Making Int J Soc Med Dec Making. 2007;27:754–61.

16. Stacey D, Bennett CL, Barry MJ, Col NF, Eden KB, Holmes-Rovner M, Llewellyn-Thomas H, Lyddiatt A, Legare F, Thomson R. Decision aids for people facing health treatment or screening decisions. Cochrane Database Syst Rev. 2011; 10:CD001431.

17. Greenfield S, Kaplan SH, Ware JE, Yano EM, Frank HJ. Patients' participation in medical care: effects on blood sugar control and quality of life in diabetes. J Gen Intern Med. 1988; 3:448–57.

18. Lin GA, Fagerlin A. Shared decision making—State of the science. Circulation: Cardiovascular Quality and Outcomes. 2014;7:328–34.

19. Benjamin EJ, Muntner P, Alonso A, Bittencourt MS, Callaway CW, Carson AP, et al. Heart disease and stroke statistics—2019 update: a report from the American heart association. Circulation. 2019;139(10):e56-528.

20. Bradley CK, Wang TY, Li S, et al. Patient-reported reasons for declining or discontinuing statin therapy: insights from the PALM registry. J Am Heart Assoc. 2019;8:e011765.

21. Fraser R, et al. Abstract Sa1076/1076. Presented at: AHA Scientific Sessions; Chicago; Nov. 10–12, 2018.

22. Eckel RH, Jakicic JM, Ard JD, de Jesus JM, Miller NH et al. 2013 AHA/ACC Guideline on Lifestyle Management to Reduce Cardiovascular Risk. A report of the American College of Cardiology/American Heart Association Task Force on Practice Guidelines. Circulation. 2014; 129: S76-S99.

23. Stone NJ, Robinson J, Lichtenstein AH, et al. 2013 ACC/AHA guideline on the treatment of blood cholesterol to reduce atherosclerotic cardiovascular risk in adults: a report of the American college of cardiology/American heart association task force on practice guidelines. J Am Coll Cardiol. 2014;63:2889–934.

24. Tobert JA. Efficacy and long-term adverse effect pattern of lovastatin. Am J Cardiol. 1988;62 (15):28J-34J.
25. Robinson J, Stone NJ. Identifying patients for aggressive cholesterol lowering: the risk curve concept. Am J Cardio. 2006;98(10):1405–8.
26. Raymond C, Cho L, Rocco M, Hazen SL. New guidelines for reduction of blood cholesterol: Was it worth the wait? Cleve Clin J Med. 2014;81(1):11–9.
27. Martin SS, Abd TT, Jones SR, Michos ED, Blumenthal RS, Blaha MJ. 2013 ACC/AHA cholesterol treatment guideline: what was done well and what could be done better. J Am Coll Cardiol. 2014;63:2674–8.
28. Pencina MJ, Navar-Boggan AM, D'Agostino RB, Williams K, Neely B, Sniderman AD, Peterson ED. Application of new cholesterol guidelines to a population-based sample. N Engl J Med. 2014;370:1422–31.
29. Nasir K, Bittencourt MS, Blaha MJ, et al. Implications of coronary artery calcium testing among statin candidates according to American College of Cardiology/American Heart Association Cholesterol Management guidelines: MESA (Multi Ethnic Study of Atherosclerosis). J Am Coll Cardiol. 2015;66:1657–68.
30. Martin SS, Sperling LS, Blaha MJ, et al. Clinician-patient risk discussion for atherosclerotic cardiovascular disease prevention: importance to implementation of the 2013 ACC/AHA Guidelines. J Am Coll Cardiol. 2015;65(13):1361–8.
31. Raza SA, Salemi JL, Zoorob RJ. Historical perspectives on prevention paradox: when the population moves as whole. J Family Med Prim Care. 2018;7(6):1163–5.
32. Rose G. Sick individuals and sick populations. Int J Epidemiol. 2001;30(3):427–32.
33. Karwalajtys T, Kaczorowski J. An integrated approach to preventing cardiovascular disease: community-based approaches, health system initiatives, and public health policy. Risk Manag Healthc Policy. 2010;3:39–48.
34. Mozzaffarian D, Benajmin EJ, Go AS, Arnett DK et al. Heart disease and stroke statistics—2016 update. A report from the American Heart Association. Circulation. 2016; 133:e38–369.
35. Goff DC Jr, Lloyd-Jones DM, Bennett G, et al. 2013 ACC/AHA guideline on the assessment of cardiovascular risk: a report of the American college of cardiology/American heart association task force on practice guidelines. Circulation. 2014;129:S49-73.
36. Montori VM, Brito JP, Murad MH. The optimal practice of evidence-based medicine: incorporating patient preferences in practice guidelines. JAMA. 2013;310:2503–4.
37. Barry MJ, Edgman-Levitan S. Shared decision making–pinnacle of patient-centered care. N Engl J Med. 2012;366:780–1.
38. Oshima Lee E, Emanuel EJ. Shared decision making to improve care and reduce costs. N Engl J Med. 2013;368:6–8.
39. Eckel RH, Jakicic JM, Ard JD, et al. 2013 AHA/ACC guideline on lifestyle management to reduce cardiovascular risk: a report of the American college of cardiology/American heart association task force on practice guidelines. J Am Coll Cardiol. 2014;63:2960–84.
40. Ropeik D. Understanding factors of risk perception. Nieman Reports. Accessed 25 Jan 2020.
41. Brown VJ. Risk perception: it's personal. Environ Health Perspect. 2014;122(10):A276–9.
42. Navar AM, Stone NJ, Martin SS. What to say and how to say it: effective communication for cardiovascular disease prevention. Curr Opin Cardiol. 2016;31(5):537–44.
43. Veldwijk J, Essers BAB, Lambooij MS, Dirksen CD, et al. Survival or mortality: Does risk attribute framing influence decision-making behavior in a discrete choice experiment? Value in Health. 2016;19(2):202–9.
44. Tversky A, Kahneman D. The framing of decisions and the psychology of choice. Science. 1981;211(4481):453–8.
45. Mayo Clinic. Statin/Aspirin Choice Decision Aid. 2013 Jul 13. https://statindecisionaid. mayoclinic.org/. Accessed 17 Dec 2019.
46. Zipkin DA, Umscheid CA, Keating NL, et al. Evidence-based risk communication: a systematic review. Ann Intern Med. 2014;161:270–80.
47. Triant VA, Perez J, Regan S, et al. Cardiovascular risk prediction functions underestimate risk in HIV infection. Circulation. 2018;137:2203–14.

48. Dalton JE, Perzynski AT, Zidar DA, et al. Accuracy of cardiovascular risk prediction varies by neighborhood socioeconomic position: a retrospective cohort study. Ann Intern Med. 2017;167:456–64.
49. DeFilippis AP, Young R, Carrubba CJ, et al. An analysis of calibration and discrimination among multiple cardiovascular risk scores in a modern multiethnic cohort. Ann Intern Med. 2015;162:266–75.
50. Lloyd-Jones DM, Braun LT, Ndumele CE, Smith SC Jr, Sperling LS, Virani SS, Blumenthal RS. Use of risk assessment tools to guide decision-making in the primary prevention of atherosclerotic cardiovascular disease: a special report from the American heart association and American college of cardiology. Circulation. 2019 Jun 18;139(25):e1162–e1177.
51. Dzaye O, Dudum R, Reiter-Brennan C, et al. Coronary artery calcium scoring for individualized cardiovascular risk estimation in important patent subpopulations after the 2019 AHA/ACC primary prevention guidelines. Prog Cardiovasc Dis. 2019;62(5):423–30.
52. Greenland P, Blaha MJ, Budoff MJ, Erbel R, Watson KE. Coronary calcium score and cardiovascular risk. J Am Coll Cardiol. 2018;72(4):434–47. https://doi.org/10.1016/j.jacc.2018.05.027.
53. Dudum R, Dzaye O, Mirbolouk M, et al. Coronary artery calcium scoring in low risk patients with family history of coronary heart disease: Validation of the SCCT guideline approach in the coronary artery calcium consortium. J Cardiovasc Comput Tomogr. 2019;13(3):21–5.
54. Budoff MJ, Young R, Burke G, et al. Ten-year association of coronary artery calcium with atherosclerotic cardiovascular disease (ASCVD) events: the multi-ethnic study of atherosclerosis (MESA). Eur Heart J. 2018;39(25):2401–8. https://doi.org/10.1093/eurheartj/ehy217.
55. Detrano D, Guerci AD, Carr JJ, et al. Coronary calcium as a predictor of coronary events in four racial or ethnic groups. N Engl J Med. 2008;358:1336–45.
56. Sarwar A, Shaw LJ, Shapiro MD, et al. Diagnostic and prognostic value of absence of coronary artery calcification.
57. Dzaye O, Dardari ZA, Cainzos-Achirica M, et al. Warranty period of a calcium score of zero: comprehensive analysis from the multiethnic study of atherosclerosis. JACC Cardiovasc Imaging. 2020. https://doi.org/10.1016/j.jcmg.2020.06.048. Epub ahead of print.
58. Mamudu HM, Paul TK, Veeranki SP, Budoff M. The effects of coronary artery calcium screening on behavioral modification, risk perception, and medication adherence among asymptomatic adults: a systematic review. Atherosclerosis. 2014;236:338–50.
59. Nasir K, McClelland RL, Blumenthal RS, et al. Coronary artery calcium in relation to initiation and continuation of cardiovascular preventive medications: the Multi-Ethnic Study of Atherosclerosis (MESA). Circ Cardiovasc Qual Outcomes. 2010;3:228–35.
60. Gupta A, Lau E, Varshney R, et al. The identification of calcified coronary plaque is associated with initiation and continuation of pharmacological and lifestyle preventive therapies: a systematic review and meta-analysis. JACC Cardiovasc Imaging. 2017;10:833–42.
61. Salami JA, Warraich H, Valero-Elizondo J, et al. National trends in statin use and expenditures in the US adult population from 2002 to 2013: insights from the medical expenditure panel survey. JAMA Cardiol. 2017;2:56–65.
62. Newman CB et al. Statin safety and associated adverse events: a scientific statement from the American heart association. Arterioscler Thromb Vasc Biol. 2019 Feb;39:e38.
63. Cannon CP, et al. Ezetimibe added to statin therapy after acute coronary syndromes. New England J Med. 2015;375(25):2387–97.
64. Robinson JG, et al. Efficacy and safety of alirocumab in reducing lipids and cardiovascular events. New England J Med. 2015;372(16):1489–99.
65. Bhatt DL, et al. Cardiovascular risk reduction with Icosapent Ethyl for hypertriglyceridemia. N Engl J Med. 2019;380:11–22.
66. Ballantyne CM, Banach M, Mancini GBJ, Lepor NE, Hanselman JC, Zhao X, Leiter LA. Efficacy and safety of bempedoic acid added to ezetimibe in statin-intolerant patients with hypercholesterolemia: a randomized, placebo-controlled study. Atherosclerosis. 2018 Oct;277:195–203.

67. Laufs U, Banach M, Mancini GBJ, Gaudet D, Bloedon LT, Sterling LR, Kelly S, Stroes ESG. Efficacy and safety of bempedoic acid in patients with hypercholesterolemia and statin intolerance. J Am Heart Assoc. 2019 Apr 2;8(7):e011662.
68. Goldberg AC, Leiter LA, Stroes ESG, Baum SJ, Hanselman JC, Bloedon LT, Lalwani ND, Patel PM, Zhao X, Duell PB. Effect of bempedoic acid vs placebo added to maximally tolerated statins on low-density lipoprotein cholesterol in patients at high risk for cardiovascular disease: the CLEAR wisdom randomized clinical trial. JAMA. 2019 Nov 12;322(18):1780–8.
69. Ray KK, Bays HE, Catapano AL, Lalwani ND, Bloedon LT, Sterling LR, Robinson PL, Ballantyne CM. CLEAR Harmony Trial. Safety and Efficacy of Bempedoic Acid to Reduce LDL Cholesterol. N Engl J Med. 2019 Mar 14;380(11):1022–1032.
70. Ballantyne CM, Laufs U, Ray KK, Leiter LA, Bays HE, Goldberg AC, Stroes ES, MacDougall D, Zhao X, Catapano AL. Bempedoic acid plus ezetimibe fixed-dose combination in patients with hypercholesterolemia and high CVD risk treated with maximally tolerated statin therapy. Eur J Prev Cardiol. 2020 Apr;27(6):593–603.
71. Esperion Therapeutics. Evaluation of major cardiovascular events in patients with, or at high risk for, cardiovascular disease who are statin intolerant treated with bempedoic acid (ETC-1002) or placebo (CLEAR Outcomes). 2016. Available at: https://clinicaltrials.gov/ct2/show/NCT02993406. Accessed 26 Oct 2020.
72. Markham A. Bempedoic acid: first approval. Drugs. 2020 May;80(7):747–753.
73. Mora S, Manson JE. Aspirin for primary prevention of atherosclerotic cardiovascular disease: advances in diagnosis and treatment. JAMA Intern Med. 2016;176:1195–204.
74. Steering Committee of the Physicians' Health Study Research Group. Final report on the aspirin component of the ongoing Physicians' Health Study. N Engl J Med 1989;321:129–35.
75. Thrombosis prevention trial. randomised trial of low-intensity oral anticoagulation with warfarin and low-dose aspirin in the primary prevention of ischaemic heart disease in men at increased risk. Lancet. 1998;351:233–41.
76. Hansson L, Zanchetti A, Carruthers SG, et al. Effects of intensive blood-pressure lowering and low-dose aspirin in patients with hypertension: principal results of the Hypertension Optimal Treatment (HOT) randomised trial. HOT Study Group Lancet. 1998;35:1755–62.
77. US Preventive Services Task Force. Aspirin for the primary prevention of cardiovascular events: recommendation and rationale. Ann Intern Med. 2002;136:157–60.
78. US Preventive Services Task Force. Aspirin for the prevention of cardiovascular disease: U.S. Preventive Services Task Force recommendation statement. Ann Intern Med. 2009;150:396–404.
79. Xie M, et al. Aspirin for primary prevention of cardiovascular events: meta-analysis of randomized controlled trials and subgroup analysis by sex and diabetes status. PLoS ONE 2014;9(10):e90286.
80. Halvorsen S, Andreotti F, et al. Aspirin therapy in primary cardiovascular disease prevention: a position paper of the European Society of Cardiology working group on thrombosis. JACC. 2014;64(3):319–27.
81. ASCEND Study Collaborative Group, Bowman L, Mafham M, Wallendszus K, Stevens W, Buck G, Barton J, Murphy K, Aung T, Haynes R, Cox J, Murawska A, Young A, Lay M, Chen F, Sammons E, Waters E, Adler A, Bodansky J, Farmer A, McPherson R, Neil A, Simpson D, Peto R, Baigent C, Collins R, Parish S, Armitage J. Effects of Aspirin for Primary Prevention in Persons with Diabetes Mellitus. N Engl J Med. 2018 Oct 18;379(16):1529–39.
82. Gaziano JM, Brotons C, Coppolecchia R, Cricelli C, Darius H, Gorelick PB, Howard G, Pearson TA, Rothwell PM, Ruilope LM, Tendera M, Tognoni G; ARRIVE Executive Committee. Use of aspirin to reduce risk of initial vascular events in patients at moderate risk of cardiovascular disease (ARRIVE): a randomised, double-blind, placebo-controlled trial. Lancet. 2018 Sep 22;392(10152):1036–46.
83. McNeil JJ, Wolfe R, Woods RL, Tonkin AM, Donnan GA, Nelson MR, Reid CM, Lockery JE, Kirpach B, Storey E, Shah RC, Williamson JD, Margolis KL, Ernst ME, Abhayaratna WP, Stocks N, Fitzgerald SM, Orchard SG, Trevaks RE, Beilin LJ, Johnston CI,

Ryan J, Radziszewska B, Jelinek M, Malik M, Eaton CB, Brauer D, Cloud G, Wood EM, Mahady SE, Satterfield S, Grimm R, Murray AM; ASPREE investigator group. Effect of aspirin on cardiovascular events and bleeding in the healthy elderly. N Engl J Med. 2018 Oct 18;379(16):1509–18.

84. Arnett DK, Blumenthal RS, et al. ACC/AHA guideline on the primary prevention of cardiovascular disease: executive summary. A report of the American college of cardiology/American heart association task force on clinical practice guidelines. J Am Coll Cardiol. 2019; 74(10)

85. Cainzos-Achirica M, Miedema MD, McEvoy JW, et al. Coronary artery calcium for personalized allocation of aspirin in primary prevention of cardiovascular disease in 2019: the MESA study (Multi-Ethnic Study of Atherosclerosis). Circulation. 2020 May 12;141 (19):1541–1553.

86. Whelton PK, et al. 2017 ACC/AHA/AAPA/ABC/ACPM/AGS/APhA/ASH/ASPC/NMA/ PCNA Guideline for the prevention, detection, evaluation, and management of high blood pressure in adults: a report of the American College of cardiology/American heart association task force on clinical practice guidelines. J Am C Cardiol. 2018;71(6):e127–248.

87. The Sprint Research Group. A randomized trial of intensive versus standard blood-pressure control. N Engl J Med. 2015;373:2103–16.

88. January CT, et al. 2019 AHA/ACC/HRS focused update of the 2014 AHA/ACC/HRS guideline for the management of patients with atrial fibrillation: a report of the American college of cardiology/American heart association task force on clinical practice guidelines and the heart rhythm society in collaboration with the society of thoracic surgeons. Circulation. 2019;140(2):e125–51.

89. Pisters R, Lane DA, et al. A novel user-friendly score (HAS-BLED) to assess 1-year risk of major bleeding in patients with atrial fibrillation. The Euro Heart Survey Chest. 2010;138 (5):1093–100.

90. Lip GY, Frison L, Halperin JL, Lane DA. Comparative validation of a novel risk score for predicting bleeding risk in anticoagulated patients with atrial fibrillation: The HAS-BLED (Hypertension, Abnormal Renal/Liver Function, Stroke, Bleeding History or Predisposition, Labile INR, Drugs/Alcohol Concomitantly) score. J Am Coll Cardiol. 2011;57(2):173080.

Index

© Springer Nature Switzerland AG 2021

S. S. Martin (ed.), *Precision Medicine in Cardiovascular Disease Prevention*,
https://doi.org/10.1007/978-3-030-75055-8

Made in the USA
Las Vegas, NV
03 June 2026

48121417R00116